Revitalized

A Guidebook to Following Your Healing Heartline

Andrea Austin, MD

Andrea Austin

Copyright © 2024

PRAISE FOR REVITALIZED

Thank you, Dr. Austin, for sharing your story and this gift to our colleagues and the wider healthcare community. *Revitalized* is a powerful testament to the courage, resilience, and innovation required to drive meaningful change. You have beautifully woven together the personal, professional, and truly practical to produce an inspiring and insightful manual for leading first self and then others. It is an essential read for the healthcare transformational leaders and changemakers of today and tomorrow.

Dr. Cheryl Martin, host of The Mind Full Medic podcast

Revitalized is an emergency physician's deeply authentic memoir from the wasteland of over-functioning, sexism, trauma, heartbreak, and burnout that can be so prevalent for women in medicine. Though the pain points are searing at times, Dr. Austin shows readers the path to revitalization, healing, and reclamation of hope and mission. This book is a masterclass in how to heal, lean into authentic self-care, and rekindle the sense of purpose that tugged you to healthcare in the first place.

Brad Johnson, PhD and David Smith, PhD, authors of Athena Rising and Good Guys

Andrea has opened her heart and her journey as a cautionary tale but also a journey of healing for all doctors. It is a must-read for physicians in the field, especially those in emergency medicine. It is packed with content and resources to guide a doctor's heart and mind.

Amanda B. Hill, JD, CEO of Guard My Practice

Dr. Andrea Austin advocates for a more supportive healthcare culture where medical providers and their colleagues can, in her words, "reclaim purpose and fulfillment within the medical profession." This is no small task, yet Dr. Austin's compelling story, keen insights, and tireless advocacy for her colleagues and the profession she loves are nothing short of an inspiration. Coupled with her podcast, "*Heartline: Changemaking in Healthcare,*" Dr. Austin is already making headway in achieving her overarching goals of revitalizing our beleaguered and labyrinthine healthcare system and the professionals who make its ponderous, yet all too necessary, wheels turn.

Keith Carlson, BSN, RN, NC-BC, host of The Nurse Keith Show

I'm not a doctor. But since I retired from the Army, I've had the distinct honor of working with them, getting to know them, and helping them understand their role as leaders. Dr Andrea Austin has penned a magnificent work that provides empathy built on experience, insight based on her scar tissue, and recommendations in a selfless (and awesome) approach to helping others navigate the extremely tough path of being a healthy and grounded physician. All healthcare professionals should read...I'm glad I did!

Lieutenant General (retired) Mark Hertling, DBA

Dr. Austin has given us a courageous, bold, and brave account of her life and work. Let us learn lessons from this book about how the heart and mind can teach us to overcome obstacles and better support one another on our life journeys.

Sheri Dewan M.S., M.D, FAANS, FCNS. Author of "Cutting a Path"

Revitalized

Dr. Austin's book is such a welcome addition to breaking down the stigma of mental health in the medical field. So often, the focus on an 'either I have it, or I don't' is such an impediment to growth and understanding of mental health. Dr. Austin's honest and vulnerable journey, as she reveals in her book, shows that mental health is a long and involved process. A long time ago, I received advice from a mentor who stated, "The thing that makes us want to be a caregiver makes us a horrible caregiver." I appreciate Dr. Austin's willingness to show how her upbringing has influenced her journey and how she has used her experiences, good and bad, to become the physician and human she initially started out to be so long ago. Her practical advice, approach to her work in a meaningful way, and creative, scientific approach make this a great read for any physician and mental health professional working with physicians.

Darren A Smith, MA LMFT, Wellness Director

The vulnerability with which Dr. Austin approaches the humanity of doctoring is so refreshing. She examines the field of medicine and its impact on those on the front lines of healing. She provides a healthy dose of empathy, normalizing the pride and heartbreak of being a healer while providing concrete tools and resources for physicians to take care of themselves to better care for others. It is a must-read for doctors, those who work with doctors, and those who are cared for by doctors.

Tiffany Mehling, MA, LCWS, Founder, Psychotherapist, Peak Performance Consultant at Persist Psych

You grow as a leader by facing your vulnerability. Dr Austin shows this beautifully by sharing her journey as a Naval ER doctor. I admire her courage and for sharing her ample resources to revitalize. I share her lifelong love for our profession and her peers, who are doctors. Thank you, Andrea, for showing us your heartline and making us stronger. May many be as inspired as I was since the very first line reading REVITALIZING.

Dr. Verena Voelter, CEO: 5P Health Care Solutions.
Author of "It Takes 5 to Tango, from Competition to
Cooperation in Health Care"

Revitalized is a compelling and deeply personal exploration of the challenges faced by healthcare professionals, particularly women in medicine. Through a blend of candid anecdotes and professional insights, Austin addresses critical issues such as burnout, gender bias, and moral injury. The book advocates for systemic changes and offers practical strategies for cultivating resilience, well-being, and compassion in the healthcare industry. Austin's narrative serves as both a memoir and a call to action, making it a poignant and essential read for anyone in the medical field.

Rajeev Kurapati MD, MBA. Author of "Burnout in Healthcare"

Revitalized by Dr. Andrea Austin underscores the profound impact of personal well-being on a clinician's ability to provide the highest quality of care. She advocates for the integration of healthcare simulation into the training regimen of providers, highlighting its transformative power in enhancing both competence and confidence. This, in turn, serves as a potent antidote to burnout, fostering a more resilient and effective healthcare workforce. Dr. Austin contributes a meaningful perspective to the ongoing discourse on healthcare provider wellness, offering actionable strategies that ultimately can elevate the standard of patient care.

Carmen N. Spalding, PhD, RN, CHSE-A

DEDICATION

This book is dedicated to a medical student who, after attending a lecture I gave on Gender Bias in medicine, asked, "Are you working on a book?" I sheepishly laughed and said, "I could never write a book." Thank you to that medical student who nudged this attending physician from her imposter syndrome.

I also dedicate this book to my husband, Chris Renders. He has been my biggest supporter, best friend, and true partner.

And to my parents. While I share some challenging stories from my youth, I know they did their best. Their hearts are huge, and they have diligently served their communities. I am forever grateful that they are my parents and raised me to be a courageous, caring, compassionate person and doctor.

A NOTE ABOUT THIS BOOK

In this book, I discuss experiences of sexual harassment, emotional trauma, post-traumatic stress, and suicidal ideation. If this could trigger you, feel free to place the book down when needed. Please get in touch with your support systems to process difficult emotions and trauma.

If you're a healthcare worker who needs help today, please contact these resources:

For ACEP Members, www.acep.org/wellness

From the National Alliance on Mental Illness, healthcare worker-specific resources: www.nami.org/Your-Journey/Frontline-Professionals/Health-Care-Professionals

Help is available for anyone in crisis, including thoughts of suicide, by calling 988 in the United States.

If you're a veteran living in the United States, you may call 988 and press 1 for veteran-specific help. You may also text 838255.

For global resources for physicians, please visit: https://physiciansanonymous.org/physician-suicide-prevention-resources/

This book is based on the personal experiences and reflections of the author, a physician who has faced burnout. While it aims to provide insight and share the author's journey, it is not intended as medical or psychological advice. The experiences and opinions expressed herein are solely those of the author and should not be considered a substitute for professional medical or psychological guidance.

Readers are encouraged to seek appropriate medical and psychological support from qualified professionals if they are experiencing symptoms of burnout, mental health issues, or any other health concerns. The author and publisher disclaim any liability arising directly or indirectly from the use or application of any information contained in this book.

Certain names and details related to my experiences have been changed to protect the privacy of those involved. This book is also a recollection of my experiences. I've done my best to relay the stories in a way that can result in learning and a better understanding of being a doctor and veteran.

The views expressed in this book are those of the author and do not reflect the official policy or position of the Department of the U.S. Navy, the Department of Defense, the U.S. government, or any other entity the author works for or with.

Revitalized

Page Blank Intentionally

TABLE OF CONTENTS

FORWARD

You might be wondering why medicine or doctors would need revitalising.

To work as a doctor in the 21st century is an extraordinary commitment, whichever healthcare system one works in. Individual doctors enter medical school empathic, academically bright, and ready to contribute to society positively. Incredibly, by the time they reach their intern year, many are disillusioned and wondering if they are up to the job. An Australian 2024 survey found that 93% of junior doctors were burnt out.[1] In the USA, work to bring the physician burnout rate down is making progress, from a high in 2021 of 63% to 48% in 2023.[2] Still, this is way too high to sustain any healthcare system that aims to take good care of patients.

In the late stages of the COVID-19 pandemic, doctors have taken the unprecedented step of going on strike in the UK, New Zealand, and South Korea. They seek to force change, recognising that the system is no longer working and is not sustainable. Historic numbers of doctors have continued to leave healthcare organisations across the UK, USA, Canada, and New Zealand. Doctors are retiring early and finding other ways to share their medical skills and knowledge outside mainstream healthcare.

It doesn't matter how the healthcare system in any given country is organised; the themes are the same. Medical doctors are no longer willing or able to work as they have in the past. Doctors' performance and capability are inextricably linked to their well-being. Currently, working in healthcare is frequently and significantly harmful to doctors.

COVID did not cause this situation; it brought known issues into the spotlight for all to see. As a patient advocate, I began learning about these issues in 2012. I wanted to understand more about the life of a doctor and make sense of what patients were experiencing in their interactions. What I learned resulted in my becoming a coach of doctors, which is how I came to meet Dr. Austin.

As I learned about the gaps in medical training and the pressures of medical culture, I began to understand how and why healthcare could sometimes go wrong. I could not unsee what I had seen. It was clear to me that doctors did not have all of the skills the community expected them to have, and 'the system' failed to respond to what doctors needed. This was negatively impacting patient care.

As a psychologist coach, I turned my attention to learning everything I could about being a doctor by talking to doctors, those who trained and employed them, and those who needed them most, patients and their families.

Since Canadian doctor William Osler created the first residency program at Johns Hopkins University in the 1890s, hospital doctors have given more and more of their lives—their time, effort, energy, and goodwill—to caring for others.

Dr. Andrea Austin has experienced all of this in her life as a doctor and generously shares her personal experience in *Revitalized* as she explores how we got here through the lens of her own experience as an emergency doctor. More importantly, she explains how we can respond to modern-day healthcare in ways that can revitalise the individual lives of doctors and the wider system that we all depend on.

Doctors want to help and care for people. They love the problem-solving aspects of their role. They expect to work with complexity, stretch their capacity, work long hours, and be on call. Modern medicine, however, has prioritised science and technology over the art of human connection, to the detriment of doctors and their patients.

Despite the relational nature of their work, doctors have received relatively little training in emotional intelligence, self-regulation, self-awareness, leadership, and interpersonal skills—all of which are needed to lead a team effectively, understand patients' complex lives, collaborate with them, and stay mentally fit enough to continue meeting the endless numbers of people suffering from illness, disorder, and tragedy.

The apprenticeship model of medical training provides an important safety net for patients. However, it also perpetuates skill gaps and collective blind spots from one generation of doctors to the next. It reinforces a deep hierarchy of power and dependence, ignoring conflicts of interest. Younger doctors seek to impress their superiors, who facilitate or hinder their reputations and progress into specialty training and other opportunities.

Overall, work hours and recognition for overtime have improved; however, as recently as last week, I spoke to a doctor who, just five years ago, was expected to work 40 hours a week and then be on call (within 10 minutes from the hospital) for another 85 hours a week. I cannot think of any other vocation with these expectations. Even the priests I know have a day a week off from their ministry to rest and restore.

It is accepted, no, it is expected, within medical culture, that the young doctor will dedicate their waking hours to work and study. Sleep is a luxury, and there is little regard for the usual young adult rites of passage. To become a doctor has meant to commit mind, body, and soul for a minimum of ten years, often stretching out to 15 or even more. They must sacrifice their youth and supportive family relationships, move away from home, and strive for perfection to serve the community. This is all part of what we have considered a *good doctor* to be and do.

As a psychologist who has been coaching doctors for a decade, I have witnessed hundreds of so-called good doctors across several countries suffer as they work to uphold their oath to put the patients first, to keep them safe, and to provide excellent healthcare in systems that undermine their intent. Doctors suffering from burnout, vicarious trauma, and moral injury are not able to perform at their best. They make more errors, have more patient complaints, and are more problematic for colleagues to work with. Too many of them end their pain by suicide.[3] It is an indescribable, unacceptable loss to the community in every regard.

I have had the very real, sometimes raw privilege of walking with Dr. Austin as her coach, from the edge of burnout through a number of powerful breakthroughs to where she is now—empowered as a change agent in her own life and into the broader healthcare system. She empowers others through her clinical practice and teaching, her podcast and writing, and her professional association leadership roles.

In *Revitalized,* Andrea writes about how her medical life exists within a context. She also shares her life outside of medicine to demonstrate the inextricable links between a doctor's humanity and their public-facing roles at work within the community. She shares her experiences as a trainee on the achievement treadmill that medicine promotes, in the military on tour and at home, in the emergency department, and as a medical educator in the simulation lab.

She gives us a three-dimensional view of life as a doctor, writing candidly about experiences of sexual harassment and intimidation with the same intensity and clarity as she writes of the beneficial impact of collegiality and coaching.

In this guide to healing, she offers many practical tools for developing compassion, setting clear personal boundaries, and aligning your work with your values to buffer the unrealistic expectations of working in healthcare. Then, she demonstrates how her intrapersonal work has enabled her agency. I am so inspired by Andrea's journey. She is actively creating better healthcare that nourishes and sustains her instead of damaging her, making her a better doctor in every regard.

You can also reclaim your inner power, assert your boundaries, and tap your own changemaker vein, uplifting your own life, your family, and everyone you interact with at work. Andrea shows you where to start and how to access the resources you need.

As a podcaster who has been in constant conversation with healthcare professionals for several years, Andrea has an expansive view of the medical landscape, especially what that means for women doctors. As an emerging leader in the US healthcare landscape, she demonstrates how important her internal work has been for fostering systems change. Andrea's story demonstrates the very real emotional and human life of a doctor and the power of compassion, agency, and human connection. The ripples from her work are unstoppable, and we are all the beneficiaries.

Revitalized: A Guidebook to Following Your Healing Heartline goes much further than individual empowerment. Dr. Austin implores us all to bring our own voice and energy collectively to create a much better healthcare system—one that inspires collective agency, innovation, and hope. One that is grounded in gratitude and joy, investing in the nobility of people valuing each other. Along with recognising the powerful value of practical heart-centered medicine. Lastly, the art of medicine enhances the science's impact on humans.

I have been privileged to be in conversation with Dr. Andrea Austin for several years as her coach. To read a book is to be in communication with the author. I hope you can listen closely and follow her lead.

Sharee Johnson
Founder Coaching for Doctors
Registered Psychologist, Professional Coach
Author of *The Thriving Doctor, How to be more balanced and fulfilled, working in medicine*

References:

1. www1.racgp.org.au/newsgp/professional/you-are-not-alone-call-for-action-amid-spate-of-gp

2. https://amp.theguardian.com/us-news/2023/sep/26/surgeons-suicide-doctors-physicians-mental-health

www.ons.gov.uk/aboutus/transparencyandgovernance/freedomofinformationfoi/suicidesinthemedicalprofession

3. www1.racgp.org.au/newsgp/professional/you-are-not-alone-call-for-action-amid-spate-of-gp

https://amp.theguardian.com/us-news/2023/sep/26/surgeons-suicide-doctors-physicians-mental-health

www.ons.gov.uk/aboutus/transparencyandgovernance/freedomofinformationfoi/suicidesinthemedicalprofession

INTRODUCTION

FROM WHITE COAT TO RECLAIMING OUR WHITE HAT

The White Coat ceremony is the first official moment of medical school. At most medical schools, parents, close family, and friends are invited to watch the new medical students walk across the stage and don their short white coats for the first time. The ceremony began in 1933 and was established by The Gold Foundation at Columbia University.

I remember my White Coat ceremony well. I was 22 years old and wanted to attend medical school more than anything. I remember the Hippocratic Oath being read,

"I swear to fulfill, to the best of my ability and judgment, this covenant:

I will respect the hard-won scientific gains of those physicians whose steps I walk and gladly share such knowledge as mine with those who are to follow.

I will apply, for the benefit of the sick, all measures [that] are required, avoiding those twin traps of overtreatment and therapeutic nihilism.

Revitalized

I will remember that there is an art to medicine as well as science and that warmth, sympathy, and understanding may outweigh the surgeon's knife or the chemist's drug.

I will not be ashamed to say, 'I know not,' nor will I fail to call in my colleagues when the skills of another are needed for a patient's recovery.

I will respect the privacy of my patients, for their problems are not disclosed to me so that the world may know. Most especially, must I tread with care in matters of life and death. If it is given to me to save a life, all thanks. But it may also be within my power to take a life; this awesome responsibility must be faced with great humbleness and awareness of my own frailty. Above all, I must not play God.

I will remember that I do not treat a fever chart or a cancerous growth but a sick human being whose illness may affect the person's family and economic stability. My responsibility includes these related problems if I am to care adequately for the sick.

I will prevent disease whenever I can, for prevention is preferable to cure.

I will remember that I remain a member of society, with special obligations to all my fellow human beings, those sound of mind and body, as well as the infirm.

If I do not violate this oath, may I enjoy life and art, be respected while I live, and be remembered with affection thereafter. May I always act to preserve the finest traditions of my calling, and may I long experience the joy of healing those who seek my help."[1]

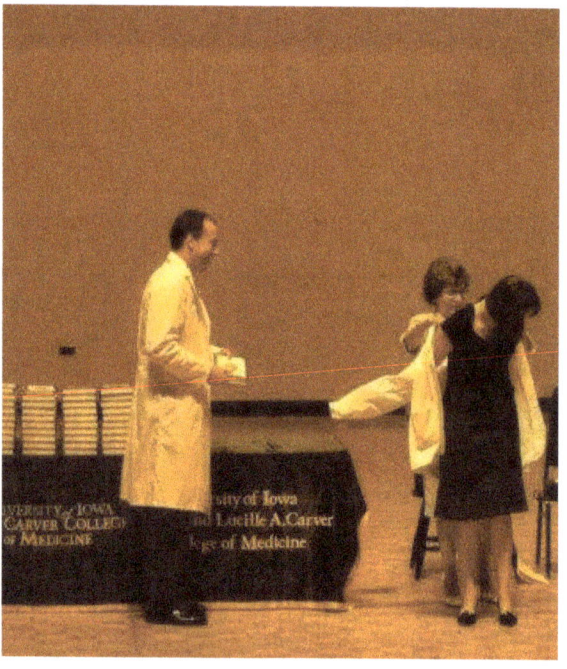

Picture of me at the White Coat Ceremony, Carver College of Medicine, August 2007.

The funny thing about the Hippocratic Oath is that I've never seen it since then.

I find it odd that this beautiful creed with all the

aspirations of a noble profession isn't hanging from the walls in all the hospitals and clinics we hurry through daily.

The system has become focused on managing the sick rather than promoting health. The art of medicine has been too often coldly extracted, and a rigid focus has been placed on the science of fixing and maximizing profits rather than the art of healing the human body and soul.

The modern version of the oath explicitly addresses the economic impact of sickness and injury on our patients. Yet, with the increasing corporatization and emphasis on profits, the healthcare system frequently takes advantage of or ignores the plight of the most economically disadvantaged patients. This dizzying and dysfunctional system has been called the "medical-industrial complex."[2] This term describes a large web of businesses, such as drug manufacturers, insurance providers, and hospital networks, that significantly influence the healthcare industry. These organizations primarily focus on making money, which can put profits before the well-being of patients and healthcare workers. This shift toward a more corporate approach, focusing on profits over patients, is problematic. Non-profit organizations are not immune either, as "no profit, no mission" encapsulates the real financial pressures that affect all payor models. The emphasis on profits, above all else, threatens both the availability and the standard of healthcare, moving us further away from the core ethical values of medicine.

This book is an invitation to rekindle the optimism and beginner's mind that doctors have when we first walk across the stage to don our white coats. The beginner's mind emphasizes dropping preconceived notions and expectations and an openness to learning and discovery.

There is a saying that the most compassionate you will be as a doctor is the start of your third year of medical school before you walk into the clinical space. We are too often resigned to the clinical space hardening student doctors. Yet, as I leave behind my hardened shell and rediscover how to connect with my heart, I find I am more empathic than on my first day of clinical medicine. I have experienced more, my heart has expanded, and thus, my capacity to heal myself, my colleagues, and my patients has grown.

To the aspiring medical students, student doctors, and hardened attendings, I admire your resilience and commitment to service. With the current challenges of our healthcare system, optimism and engaging in the work to change the system is viewed as naïve. I urge you to hold onto that light within you fiercely. Many forces within the medical-industrial complex will intentionally and unintentionally try to dim that light. Let this book serve as your guide, connecting you to that light and equipping you with the tools to navigate your journey and, if you choose, also reshape yourself and the system.

The journey to becoming a doctor is seen as a noble pursuit, a calling to heal and make a difference in the lives of others. It's a demanding path, and as a pre-medical student, the altruism coursing through my veins provided an abundant energy source.

As a pre-med student, I organized group meetings and guest speakers to enlighten us about their journeys as doctors. One such speaker stands out, not for his specialty or accolades, but for the darkness that permeated his words. Perched on the desk at the front of the room, his eyes reflected wisdom and weariness. He shared the harsh realities of his career—a relentless pursuit of success that led to long hours, a failed marriage, dwindling reimbursements, and an overwhelming lack of time with patients. His words lingered, painting a bleak picture of the profession we were preparing to enter. His words troubled me, and while my altruism was a mighty shield, I began to feel uncertain about the path ahead. Could I end up like him? I wondered if he was once a chipper pre-medical student like me.

Curiously, as I saw the etched lines on his face, I realized he seemed older than his years. Fifteen years later, in my midlife unraveling[3] during the darkest days of the pandemic, his words repeated in my mind, and regret reverberated for not heeding his warning. I sensed that my frequent furrowing and pained expressions were accelerating my wrinkles, too. While the Botox® was freezing the outward appearance of the furrows, there was no hiding from the indelible marks etched more deeply into my soul.

Those premature lines on his face were the visible representation of the impact of moral injury from doctoring in the medical-industrial complex. Moral injury, first described in soldiers, is "when one feels they have violated their conscience or moral compass when they take part in, witness or fail to prevent an act that disobeys their own moral values or personal principles."[4]

The system, once designed to care and heal, had become a convoluted maze of bureaucracy and an ever-increasing distance between doctors and patients. Many of us struggle with this after the initial excitement of being in clinical spaces fades because the truth about the weight of this burden, trying to doctor under an increasing strain of moral injury, was glossed over in the lead-up to and during medical school.

However, I refused to let go of the flickering flame, fueling my desire to practice medicine. I began to realize that the reasons I became a doctor would not be the same reasons I stayed a doctor. I had to remove the rose-colored, altruistic glasses I had when I entered medical school, and letting go of the belief that the system was broken beyond repair was required. I had to pave a new path to walk with integrity while doctoring. This new path was difficult. To stay in medicine, I must embrace a new identity as a changemaker.

There was no example of what a changemaker doctor was during medical school. Most doctors spend their days seeing patients. Now, I spend most of my time teaching, writing, and coaching doctors. This book explains my transformation to where I am fulfilled practicing medicine. Being fulfilled does not mean being happy all the time. Doctoring requires witnessing immense amounts of human suffering. Yet, as my husband reminds me nearly every day, what we do matters. Our careers, when practiced with our hearts, have the potential to be meaningful and fulfilling.

This book is not only for healthcare professionals but also for the patients who have uttered the words, "I hate my doctor." I've listened to countless family members and friends complain about curt treatment and, sometimes, devastating errors. I won't make excuses for doctors. Yet, I know there is a human within that doctor and that there is probably an explanation (not an excuse) for their behavior. The long hours and colossal patient volume with only a fraction of the time required to address their concerns are a few reasons the sacred bond between doctors and patients is frayed.

In the pages that follow, I hope my story inspires understanding and compassion. To transform our healthcare system from one that manages the sick to one that promotes healing and health, we must start by cultivating the qualities in doctors that will nurture their emotional, spiritual, and physical well-being. For example, why is it okay for your surgeon to operate on you after having not slept for 24 hours? We impose rigorous standards upon pilots to safeguard passenger safety, including insisting on appropriate levels of rest. Yet, we fail to demand the same level of commitment to patient well-being. It is time to demand change and place your safety and care at the forefront. The well-being of doctors and patients is inextricably linked.

Health encompasses many intricacies, and the doctor must unravel the threads to discern the interconnectedness of various issues. A study has shown that primary care doctors need 26.7 hours to address the work assigned to them in an average day, with three hours of inbox and documentation tasks.[5] Even if artificial intelligence (AI) algorithms can streamline many workflows, how will we ensure AI lets us reallocate that time for the human side of doctoring and not just seeing more patients to generate more revenue?[6] I am increasingly convinced that the answer begins with listening to our heartlines and asserting boundaries to care for ourselves and our patients.

This book is an empowering guide that will equip you with the tools to protect and preserve the light within you. I will share the lessons I have learned, the strategies I have discovered, and the tools I have developed to navigate this convoluted and sometimes treacherous path.

This book is a call to action for doctors to heal thyself and reclaim their white hats. For those unfamiliar with the phrase, white hat means someone acting for morally good reasons. While there are intellectual arguments and strategies for reclaiming our white hats, this book will focus on the emotional side of being a doctor and developing the skills to, as Dr. Susan David encourages, have the emotional agility to navigate these challenges.[7]

Palmistry, the art of reading palms, is not science. But I can see why people are drawn to it: It offers a glimpse into the future to answer the question I'm asked, "Will I be okay? While medicine relies on facts, there is growing evidence that compassion, connection, and emotional well-being are integral to well-being. A term from palmistry resonates deeply with me: the heartline, the horizontal crease in the palm that is said to represent our emotional nature. I am drawn to this term because, on the cerebral journey to be a doctor, I lost sight of my heartline. By reconnecting with my heartline, I found my way back to healing my patients and myself.

So many well-being books are out there, and many are marketed to physicians. What is different about this book? Physician well-being is both something from within and very much affected by external factors of our work environments, political decisions that impact funding, and even the ability to care for patients in a way we are called to by the Hippocratic Oath. While many changes are needed to improve the healthcare system, we must start with ourselves. This book will provide the life preserver you need to up your well-being to be more whole and, if you choose, engage in larger change efforts. Remember that physicians are resilient. We self-select to do some of the most emotionally challenging work, from holding the hand of the dying to breaking the news of deaths to the living. Resilience is a term that has been weaponized against physicians, especially when we speak out for changes to the system. This book provides next-level tips for well-being that are more established in other fields, such as psychotherapy, organizational psychology, and neuroscience. It applies them through the context of modern physicians' struggles. We must increase our emotional intelligence to be the leaders and changemakers the system desperately needs.

As a practical matter, the book is organized into three parts: Part One is the early years of my life, Part Two is the messy during medical school through my early attending years, and Part Three is The Revitalization, in which I weave in all I've learned about promoting emotional, physical, and spiritual well-being in doctors. There will be vignettes from my life, clinical cases, and interactions in my career that provide tangible examples of the challenges I faced and how to apply the concepts in the book. In addition, at the end of each chapter, there will be prompts that invite you to:

Reflect:

Slow down, let your mind wander, journal.

Reframe:

This involves a mindset shift. Is there another way of thinking about the topic, issue, or problem? Note I don't always include the reframe prompt. Remember, you are in charge, and you know your life best. In some cases, reframing can be too close to gaslighting ourselves, for example, asking ourselves to find a silver lining in something that is just crappy. Skip the reframe if you don't think it applies or feels good.

Reimagine:

This invitation will vary from reimagining your life to, and at times, reimagining the healthcare system. I'll encourage you to think about how to exercise your agency to improve your life and medicine. Please note, like everything in this book, do only what feels good. The first time you pick up this book, you may be burned out and need to focus inward. Later, you may want to change the system as you heal.

Respond:

This is a call to action to make positive changes in your life and career.

Resources:

Last, I'll include resources to guide your continued growth.

I love doctors. We work so hard, and doctors deserve to not merely survive medicine but thrive. This is a guidebook to rediscovering and, for those aspiring doctors, staying connected to your heartline. ~Andrea Austin, M.D.

PART 1: THE EARLY YEARS

Andrea Austin

CHAPTER 1

HYPERFUNCTIONING IN CHAOS

"Some of the things that happened to us in childhood can be reactivated by working with patients, and that these early traumas that I didn't think were that big of a deal, actually did need to be processed." — Dr. Andrea Austin, on Heartline podcast, Nov 15, 2022

We all develop coping mechanisms to get through life. I developed hyperfunctioning to navigate my childhood and, later, a strategy to deal with the stress of doctoring. Hyperfunctioning is when a part of the body goes above and beyond its usual work rate, working harder than it should. When we talk about hyperfunctioning in terms of how we think and process, it's like our minds are always on overdrive. It's as if our brains are like computers with too many apps running simultaneously, working around the clock without downtime. This state involves a lot of thinking, planning, analyzing, and worrying. When you've been hyperfunctioning for years, your nervous system rewires to a new normal, and it's difficult even to realize that it is happening.

Signs you may be hyperfunctioning: It's hard to stay still and do nothing. You have a constant to-do list; even a day off turns into a list of projects. When there is a conflict or a problem, you leap in to solve it without checking in to see if your cup is full before engaging on the issue and before others can intervene. Note that this tendency creates an atmosphere in which the more you jump in, the fewer others jump in. Eventually, this leads to resentment when no one else jumps in and continually depletes your energy.

Hyperfunctioning is a maladaptive coping mechanism. My childhood convinced me that the best way to move through the world was to take care of everything myself. Despite my parents being very loving, a baseline level of chaos permeated our home. Until I was a teenager, my mom's job required us to live at the Four-Plex. Our family occupied one of the apartments, while the other three were home to individuals with disabilities—some physical and some intellectual. My mom's role was helping them, whether grocery shopping, budgeting, or attending medical appointments. It was like living in a group home, with each person having their apartment and leading their own life. But living in such proximity permitted us to be ready to help.

In kindergarten, I belonged to the Girl Scouts, a youth organization for young girls. We met every other week, and like all six-year-olds, I couldn't keep track of on weeks or off weeks. My mom dropped me off for Girl Scouts, and I went down the stairs into the church. I suddenly realized no one was there, and it was pitch black. I ran back outside, and my mom was gone. I was there alone. Cell phones didn't exist, and I was far from home.

I figured my best option was to go back inside and try to reach the phone and call home. Thankfully, a school assignment had been to memorize our phone numbers. I still remember how scared I was trying to find my way in the dark, and then I realized I couldn't reach the phone. I was in a total panic. I ran back outside, crying, and someone recognized me.

Further adding to my panic was this was a stranger, and as a dedicated rule follower, I knew I wasn't supposed to talk to strangers. Yet, out of desperation, I followed him into the church basement to call my parents. Fortunately, he was a good person that helped summon my parents.

This story may seem trivial to an adult, yet it was terrifying. Early in life, this and a few other pivotal events taught me that trusting adults was risky. It was better to get a planner, write down everything I could, and count on myself. It is sad to think that, as a six-year-old, I began to lose trust in others. I didn't believe they could care for me or be trusted. While it seems like a minor trauma, that night in the church basement, I was terrified. I felt like I might die. While years later, I understood this was a thought distortion, my brain and body were already hard-wired that hyperfunctioning was a life-saving practice rather than the life-draining practice it is.

Later, my mom developed severe depression. When I was 12, she checked herself into a mental hospital while my dad and I were away on a camping trip. It is heart-wrenching, thinking about the shame she felt, waiting until we were out of town and possibly out of reach of phones before seeking help. I'm so grateful she had the strength and insight to ask for help.

Her initial hospitalization was brief, but once home, her depression worsened. She would spend most of her days in the dark basement, emerging only to eat a meager meal. She lost a dramatic amount of weight; it felt like we were watching her fade out from us both emotionally and physically. Agoraphobia consumed her, and I desperately hoped that getting her outside, basking in the warmth of the summer sun, would somehow cure her.

I begged her to come outside, believing that the sunlight could permeate her body and chase away the darkness that had settled within her soul. Well-intentioned, I tried pulling her onto the porch, but it only worsened things. I could see the uncontrollable shaking, the anguish in her eyes. I realized I was hurting her, not physically but emotionally. Deep down, I knew that her struggle resulted from a physiological imbalance, something beyond my control. No amount of well-meaning words or gestures could magically fix it.

With no improvement after the trial of outpatient

therapy after the first hospitalization, she was re-admitted to the psychiatric unit. This time, they kept her for what felt like an eternity—a month of intense treatment. And thankfully, she came home much improved. Witnessing her transformation as she reconnected with her body and mind was inspiring. As an avid reader, I directed my reading towards books about the brain and biology. I didn't think about being a doctor. It was more a curiosity about how the brain's neurochemicals could shift and lead to a mood disorder.

Looking back, what saddens me the most is the lack of support for my family. My dad did his best, but he was hurting, too, and we all needed support. It's a testament to the fragmented nature of our healthcare system that family therapy isn't considered an integral part of healing. I didn't receive any formal counseling or support to process what happened to my mom.

Living involves going through traumatic experiences, and physicians are exposed to large daily doses of emotional trauma. The intense experiences of doctoring reactivated some of the rough edges of my unprocessed childhood trauma. It was a friend, also a physician, who later suggested that some of us in intense specialties, like emergency medicine, may be drawn to chaos due to our chaotic upbringings.

Now, this is only true for some. Many of my colleagues had relatively normal childhoods, perhaps with fewer adverse experiences than mine. But for me, there was an unconscious attraction to drama and intense experiences—a residue of the turbulence I grew up with. And maybe that's not entirely bad. The chaos and, at times, the volume of my home strangely prepared me for the emergency department. At least initially, I didn't feel threatened by the commotion because it felt familiar, reminiscent of my own house.

Fast forward to 2017, I was an emergency medicine attending in the Navy, deployed to Kuwait after a few months in Iraq. The two experiences couldn't have been more different. Iraq was a combat zone, and we were taking care of mainly Iraqis injured by improvised explosive devices (IEDs) and gunshots. It was adrenaline-packed, and my days were busy with patient care, briefs to the base commander, and educating our medical teams. As a hyperfunctioning person, I was in my element.

When I arrived in Kuwait, most of the team I reintegrated with had been there for months. They had a rhythm for covering the clinic and other administrative duties, which was a welcome break at first. Yet, I was reliant on my hyperfunctioning- there were only so many books to read, manuscripts to write, movies to watch, and workouts to do, and soon, I began to feel worthless. Sadness, loneliness, grief, and anger began to emerge during the long nights alone.

Convinced that it was just deployment and that I'd feel better once I got home, I bottled the emotions. While there were a lot of happy moments after I returned home, a recurrent wave of anger kept bubbling up. The intensity and unpredictability were disconcerting. After years of counseling returning service members to reach out for help, I recognized that it was time for me to go to therapy.

It had been a decade since my last visit to a therapist. Back then, the sessions focused on my divorce and involved a practical, problem-solving approach to navigating the logistical hurdles of being a medical student while disentangling my personal life. We never dug into my family history or the experiences that shaped me. Thus, I felt curious and skeptical as I sat on the therapist's couch, with a box of tissues prominently placed next to me.

My initial resistance began to soften as the therapist shared her approach. She emphasized the importance of understanding my family story as the foundation of her particular form of therapy. As an emergency medicine doctor, I thrived on swift problem-solving and efficiently addressing urgent needs. Revisiting childhood experiences seemed indulgent and lacked the immediacy I craved.

Still, the therapist persisted. I watched her sketch a family tree—an outline of my parents, siblings, and their roles in my life as I spoke. Reluctantly, I shared tidbits about their professions, geographic locations, and any mental health conditions I knew about. As we traversed the branches of my family tree, we stumbled upon hidden secrets, unearthing snippets of stories that had long been forgotten. While I had thought about some things that had happened in my childhood, the power of saying them out loud helped me realize the depth of wounds resurfacing in my current life.

With the stroke of her pen, the therapist drew a circle, a visual representation of our baggage. She spoke candidly, her words mirroring my inclination toward colorful language. She called it a "bag of shit"—a collection of life's challenges, traumas, and struggles. The tactics I had tried, such as ignoring it, comparing it (my bag is smaller, less significant than others), or my favorite, ruminating on various parts but not processing it, was resulting in an overloaded bag of shit bubbling out as angry outbursts.

My childhood scored moderate for ACEs—adverse childhood experiences. It's a screening exam that explores various aspects, including physical and emotional abuse, neglect, caregiver mental illness, and household violence. Now, my childhood wasn't the worst by any means, but what we know about trauma is that our bodies and minds don't discern the gradients of its impact, especially when we're young children. Even experiences that may seem mild to some can still have a profound effect.

My childhood taught me that many patterns we establish as children are not our choices. I adapted to the topsy-turvy schedule, and later in life, when I chose a profession, I didn't question the impact of working rotating shifts, weekends, and holidays. Childhood and family dynamics frequently cause limiting beliefs, defined as beliefs we subconsciously and, at other times, consciously hold onto without definitive evidence. Through this book, I will encourage you to reflect on what limiting beliefs are holding you back.

Reflect:

What is something you assumed was how your life would be, based on your childhood, that you're ready to let go of now? Consider your personal finances, profession, who you would partner with, and where you would live. Let your mind wander on what you've always taken as a truth about how you'd live your life.

_____

_____

_____

_____

It's important to acknowledge that not all parts of my childhood were difficult. There were beautiful experiences that positively impacted my path. I grew up in Vinton, Iowa, where the Braille School, a specialized school for visually impaired students, was located. I'm thankful that students from the Braille School also attended some classes at the public schools. From a young age, as we were learning to read, they were learning to read Braille, feeling the pages and deciphering the words. It was remarkable to watch their fingers move across the pages, sometimes struggling to make sense of the words, analogous to us sounding words out. It was incredibly impactful because, at times, we could help them learn a word their fingers couldn't decipher by looking at it. The inverse occurred as well. This experience taught me the importance of service. It also helped me develop a deeper understanding of the balance of helping people with disabilities and staying curious and receptive to their unique gifts and abilities to contribute.

These experiences and values have shaped my journey as a doctor. They have taught me the importance of empathy, compassion, and the power of community. Looking back, I see how these early lessons laid the foundation for my passion for service and my dedication to improving the lives of others.

On the flip side, in the chaotic realm of my childhood home, boundaries were a foreign concept. The constant knocks on our doors, asking us for help, created a sense of accessibility that blurred the lines between our family's needs and the demands of others. The lack of boundaries in my home pre-conditioned me to accept many encroachments on boundaries as a doctor. Service was above any need to care for self, and this patterning was then easily transitioned into the concept that the patient's needs come before the physician. While during the pandemic, the phrase "put on your oxygen mask before helping others" became more mainstream as a reminder for physicians to care for themselves, it's still counter-cultural in medicine.

Let's spend a minute on the concept of the Well-being Cup. We'll get into it more in later chapters, but it's important to start connecting with your emotional and physical capacity or energy. During medical training, you are programmed to ignore your cup and encouraged to put the patient first at your peril. While rooted in service, this is a hazardous practice, as it can result in working while tired or ill, seriously draining your cup.

Reflect:

How full is your Well-being Cup (emotional and physical capacity)? Color how full your cup is right now.

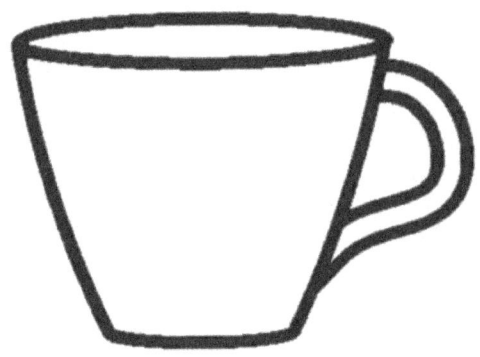

If your cup is not full, what do you need to fill it back up? Still trying to figure it out? No worries, this book will offer many ideas on what you may need to fill your cup again. During the worst phases of the pandemic, I wasn't sure what would fill my cup again. If that's where you are, that's okay. Flag this page and return to it after you read more of the book.

Write down what you need to fill your cup below:

_____

_____

_____

_____

Our apartment building was a hub of perpetual assistance. If a neighbor's toilet got clogged, my mom or dad would rush to fix it. We were there to lend a hand if the smoke detector went off. Even if a simple task like changing the batteries in a TV remote was required, we willingly stepped in. As I grew older, I actively participated in helping others in our building. There was undeniable satisfaction in being of service, and each person we assisted deserved our support. Yet, there was another side to this constant giving, one that affected the well-being of our family.

The constant tending to others outside our family occasionally affected my mother's ability to care for me. My tonsillectomy was physically painful, with an added layer of emotional trauma. I was only five or six years old, and waking up from the surgery, I felt an unbearable pain in my throat. It was excruciating. But instead of the comfort and reassurance of my mother's presence, she chose to focus on one of her clients, taking them grocery shopping or some other activity. Alone in the hospital, unable to speak due to the pain, I remember the phone ringing—a concerned relative trying to check on me. The silence in my throat mirrored the anger and sadness that overwhelmed me. I longed for my mother's support, and the absence of it fueled a deep sense of abandonment.

While our bustling household offered excitement and a sense of purpose, it came at a cost. After venting about these experiences, my husband reminds me that these very circumstances shaped me into the capable person I am today. Undoubtedly, I have the self-reliance and resilience that comes from being a self-starter from a young age. It requires ongoing work to channel the adaptive aspects of our strengths and manage the maladaptive tendencies. Note I didn't say let go; they're always there. Yet, with neuroplasticity, these well-worn pathways in our brain can become less automatic, and we can fast-track the adaptive circuits.

Digging into our family origin stories and unlocking the attachments and behaviors influenced by our upbringing can yield profound insights into our present lives. While many of us are taught to "leave the past in the past," scientific evidence supports the impact of our childhood experiences on our relationships and behaviors. Recognizing this, I later underwent Eye Movement Desensitization and Reprocessing therapy (EMDR). We'll discuss what EMDR is and how it may help you later in the book. Together, my therapist and I focused on revisiting pivotal moments from my childhood, processing the emotions and stories, and reshaping the narratives tied to them to be more aligned with an authentic and inspiring way to move forward.

Through this therapeutic journey, I began to experience a profound shift in my life, positively affecting my roles as a wife, a doctor, and an individual navigating this world. Adopting a growth mindset and self-compassion began to contract the profound wounds of my childhood considerably, and I later became a veteran and doctor. I hope this book serves as a window into the hidden layers of our beings, shedding light on what lies beneath the surface.

Reflect:

What is a hurt from your childhood that continues to show up negatively in your life now?

_____

_____

_____

_____

Reframe:

While nothing can be done to erase the hurt, is there anything you need now to process this hurt?

_____
_____
_____

_____

Respond:

Is there an action you want to take to address unhelpful patterns from childhood? A few ideas to get started: read a book, talk with a friend, or find a therapist. Also, there is an emerging trend of adult children undergoing therapy with their adult parents. In an interview on Glennon Doyle's podcast (*We Can Do Hard Things*, episode 247) about her memoir, *Thicker Than Water*, Kerry Washington shares that therapy with her adult parents following a family secret being revealed helped the entire family heal.

_____
_____
_____

_____

Reimagine:

How can understanding family dynamics and systems enhance a doctor's empathy toward patients and their families?

_____

_____

_____

_____

Resources:

The Body Keeps the Score: Brain, Mind, and Body in the Healing of Trauma by Bessel van der Kolk is viewed as one of the foundational books on the impact of emotional trauma on our minds and bodies. In the last third of the book, we'll cover more about trauma and recovery.

Disentangling from Emotionally Immature People by Lindsay C. Gibson. Many of our parents did their best with what they knew and had at the time. Now, going to therapy is much more commonplace. This book helps you reconnect with your inner child and meet her needs today as an adult.

Military One Source is a service the Department of Defense provides for 24/7 confidential help, information, and resources. Their website is www.militaryonesource.mil/ or call 800-342-9647.

Vet Centers are community-based counseling centers. www.vetcenter.va.gov/

If this chapter stirred something in you that you want to unpack with a therapist, and you're not sure how to find a therapist, this article provides tips to get started: www.healthline.com/health/how-to-find-a-therapist-our-tips

Learn more about Adverse Childhood events from www.cdc.gov/violenceprevention/aces/index.html. I also highly recommend *What Happened to You* by Dr. Bruce Perry and Oprah.

Andrea Austin

CHAPTER 2

NAVIGATING NOW: INSIGHTS FROM YOUR PAST

"I gave up good to go to great. Don't settle for anything less than what fulfills you." —Dr. Amy Vertrees on Heartline podcast, Oct 17, 2023

I am the only doctor in my family. While things were sometimes hectic at home, school became a welcome area of stability. I loved reading. My half-brother is six years older than me, and my half-sister is about 12 years older than me. They only visited during the summers, so I spent much time alone after school. Reading opened me up to new places and expanded my mind.

Even from a young age, I didn't fit in with other kids. My mom frequently took me to dinners with her friends, and I got used to either talking with the grown-ups or reading on my own.

I loved learning and strongly desired to please my teachers. Looking back, I think that's when my people-pleasing and perfectionism began. Getting in trouble, missing an answer on a test, or anything "bad" was to be avoided at all costs. While I didn't know what I wanted to do with my life, I sensed that being smart was essential and would open up doors for me.

My fifth-grade teacher recognized that I struggled with perfectionism. She often said, "Your best will do just fine." That saying never worked for me, and it was not until many years later, while reading *The Perfectionist's Guide to Losing* Control by Katherine Morgan Schafler, that I figured out why it bothered me so much. Our best isn't always fine. It's not a true statement. There can be real consequences when our best misses the mark, especially while doctoring. If I miss intubation, the patient could die or sustain a brain injury due to oxygen deprivation.

Now, I don't say my best will do just fine. I have a framework that rings true for me and can be called on when my perfectionism crosses into maladaptive territory. First, I step back and assess if a task requires a perfect performance. There are times when near perfection is required. These are rare moments, and knowing the difference has dramatically added to my energy reserve. For years, I was demanding perfection from myself and those around me (for all of you, my sincerest apologies), which was an unsustainable way to live and work. When I determine that less than perfection is acceptable, I will coach myself to put in 80% effort. I've found that my 80% is usually still a good showing and rarely draws criticism.

My first interest in medicine was going to the doctor.

There was a physician assistant in my hometown, Becky. I enjoyed talking with her and was amazed by the fast and kind way she solved problems. In sixth grade, we had the opportunity to participate in "Take Our Daughters to Work Day." I asked if I could shadow Becky instead of a parent. Thankfully, everyone agreed. I spent the day following her from room to room, listening to interesting stories and Becky doing the detective work to solve the medical mystery. I enjoyed connecting with people and integrating that with the science of medicine. I was hooked.

I was 13 years old when the McCaughey septuplets were born in Des Moines, IA. While it might not sound as noteworthy today, this was a monumental medical achievement. Dr. Paula Mahone and Dr. Karen Drake were the perinatologists who delivered the babies. There was a media blitz around these deliveries. In a state 90% White, seeing two Black women doctors featured on the cover of magazines and TV was inspiring. I wrote Dr. Mahone a letter and shared my desire to be a doctor with her, and I also requested to shadow her. I met Dr. Mahone and Dr. Drake in their Des Moines clinic a few months later.

Dr. Mahone shared her experiences of racism and sexism in medicine. She didn't sugarcoat it. She also instilled in me that you could be a caring woman doctor. As a perinatologist, she gave bad news to a lot of women and families, including miscarriages and stillbirths. I asked her how she dealt with these tragedies. She said that she occasionally cried alongside her patients. That's when I had a feeling that I could be a doctor.

I recognize that I am an "empath." I feel others' emotions intensely. I am an emotional person. This began in childhood, with early memories of tearing up at somber songs. I was worried this would prevent me from being a doctor, as I knew my empathy would be hard to manage. Hearing Dr. Mahone explain that I could show some emotions helped me feel like maybe I could be a doctor. Later, a medical school professor shared, "You can cry with your patients. Just don't be crying so hard they have to console you."

That ability to feel the emotion without being consumed by it has been a journey I'm still on. I recall a recent patient who presented with cardiac arrest. As we worked to resuscitate him, a nurse walked in, and she said, "That's my dad." This nurse had been particularly kind to me in my first few months working at our hospital. She was competent and a strong leader. Seeing her crying and overcome with emotion created a powerful wave of emotions in me. I felt the tears well and didn't fight them; I knew she saw them too. I said, "I'm so sorry. We're doing our best right now." My voice cracked. We hugged, and I got back to work on the resuscitation.

There was a moment when I felt the tears, and I thought, *"You're not strong enough for this after all these years, and you still cry sometimes."* I realized that the old, patriarchal style of medicine still wells up in me on occasion. I am strong because I show up, *especially* because I will be vulnerable enough to tear up with my team, patients, and family. And I keep showing up, even though it can sometimes be so painful.

In high school, I had a science teacher who was far from my favorite teacher, at least early on. He was exacting, and I spent a lot of time on homework for his chemistry classes. Yet, he was motivating. He encouraged me to apply for a full scholarship to a nearby university. The scholarship required taking an exam. He encouraged me to take the chemistry exam. I told him that I'd take the biology exam instead. He tried to persuade me to take the chemistry exam, as he felt that the chemistry classes had been more challenging and that I was more prepared for that exam. I listened to my gut, and I took the biology exam. I got the full ride. I learned a valuable lesson I would have to relearn a few more times: It is good to take the counsel of others, especially those more experienced, but you know your life. You have to make the choices, especially when they're high stakes. Ultimately, you can make the best decisions when you're in touch with your true desires and have insights into your strengths and limitations. I am proud of the 17-year-old Andrea, who wouldn't be swayed too easily and listened to herself.

Reflecting on Becky and Dr. Mahone taught me the power of networking and mentoring. None of us can do anything challenging without support. While my parents were loving and caring, they knew little about the journey to becoming a doctor. Becky and Dr. Mahone showed me how to get into medical school through shadowing and mentorship.

I am also thankful to Becky's nurse, Michelle Burns. She is now a physician assistant (PA). I asked Michelle if I should be a PA or a doctor. Michelle looked at me and said, "Andrea, you have the time and the ability to become a doctor. Go to medical school." That stuck with me. Those words steadied me many times.

In many cases, we minimize our impact on others. To this day, the best moments for me are when I'm mentoring or coaching a pre-med medical student, resident, or fellow attending. Medicine is hard. None of us do it alone. Reaching out and helping each other is vital to enhancing our fulfillment.

Mentorship is a guiding force for those navigating the maze-like corridors of medicine. Mentoring acts as a compass, providing aspiring doctors with essential direction as they navigate the complexities of their chosen path. By offering invaluable insights and guidance, mentorship empowers them to overcome the inevitable challenges and hurdles they will encounter.

Mentorship's impact goes beyond the immediate mentee-mentor relationship. It radiates outward, generating a ripple effect of care, compassion, and support. As mentees flourish under their mentors' guidance, they become a source of inspiration for others, embodying the values instilled within them and later becoming mentors to others.

Thus, mentorship becomes a virtuous cycle, perpetuating a culture of learning, growth, and mutual support. By embracing the role of mentorship, we not only invest in the personal and professional development of others but also contribute to the overall well-being of the medical community. Within this interconnected web of mentorship, individuals can thrive, and the collective spirit of caring can flourish.

In this ongoing journey of mentorship, let us harmonize our efforts, nurturing a community that uplifts, sustains, and empowers one another. By investing in the growth and well-being of those around us, we contribute to a stronger, more resilient medical community built on collaboration, compassion, and camaraderie.

This chapter's title is Navigating Now: Insights From Your Past. Reflecting on why we become doctors can help channel the beginner's mind and rediscover the awe and excitement of practicing medicine.

No one person can be your everything. In residency, I recognized this and began cultivating mentors for various personal and professional development aspects. For example, I had mentors I reached out to hone my clinical acumen, another for leadership direction, and a few that helped me navigate the gender dynamics of doctoring.

Reflect:

Please reflect on why you became a healthcare professional.

_____

_____

Who were the important people who helped you become a healer along the way?

_____

_____

_____

Have you let them know?

_____

_____

_____

Respond:

When you think about why you became a healthcare

professional, do those reasons still resonate with you? Why or why not?

_____

_____

_____

Reimagine:

We all need mentors and sponsors throughout our careers, including after training, when we may face periods of burnout, boredom, or setbacks. How does your workplace promote mentoring, sponsoring, and coaching? Is there a way to make it more accessible?

_____

_____

_____

Andrea Austin

CHAPTER 3

CAMARADERIE AND COMPASSION: EARLY JOBS AND THE GROWTH OF EMPATHY

"It's the person you are becoming on the way to your goal. That is the secret sauce and smelling the flowers." — Dr. Amanda Dinsmore, Heartline podcast Jan 2, 2024

My first employment experience involved working at the concession stand at Moose's Rollerina in Vinton, Iowa. The proprietors, Moose and Marion, proved to be exceptional bosses, exhibiting kindness, fairness, and flexibility in scheduling my shifts. It felt like a dream job for a 14-year-old who wanted to spend time at the skating rink, complete with free entry and a complimentary snack at the end of each shift!

As time progressed, I worked my way up to becoming a DJ at the roller rink, a role that I unabashedly consider the coolest job I've ever had (only half-joking here). This position granted me the authority to select the music and wield a whistle to enforce Rollerina rules. Learning to skate backward became a favorite skill, especially during the themed backward skate sessions where I could blow my whistle to command a change in skating direction.

Additionally, the hokey pokey on skates added an extra layer of challenge compared to its foot-based counterpart, making for an enjoyable and sometimes hilarious experience.

I regret not prolonging my tenure as a DJ, a position I resigned from as my interest in medicine deepened. I shifted my focus toward becoming a certified nursing assistant (CNA), exploring the fundamentals of helping with a healthcare setting, primarily within a nursing home. The absence of my paternal grandparents, who passed away before or during my early years, left a void, and I had limited memories of my maternal grandparents due to their declining health when I was still relatively young. Working in the nursing home allowed me to establish connections with older individuals and explore my interest in healthcare.

Among the residents, Jim became my favorite resident to visit. A retired farmer, Jim wore overalls every day. He was kind, soft-spoken, and an avid reader like me. During the mid-mornings or mid-afternoons, I would bring around the water cart and converse with him about a book or the weather (always a good conversation starter in the Midwest). Over the subsequent years, I saw Jim grapple with increasing difficulty walking and spending more time confined to his room. Then, one day, I received the news of his passing during the previous night. Visiting his room one last time to bid farewell, I questioned whether I was suited for a medical career. The challenge of forming deep connections, only to face the pain of loss, left me wondering how I would endure losing patients of my own one day.

In addition to the sorrow accompanying the decline and eventual passing of the residents, there were troubling parts of my experience working in the nursing home. One glaring observation was the financial struggle experienced by most of the CNAs employed there. For many, this job wasn't viewed as a calling but perceived as the best option among a pool of less-than-ideal employment opportunities. Each morning, we received a list of the residents we needed to help get ready. Although my memory has faded, I recall the list comprising six residents. With an average of 10-15 minutes assigned for each person, the only viable approach was to rush and cut corners. Struggling to complete my list, I would bring a resident a few minutes late to breakfast. Looking back, I discerned that I was experiencing moral injury even as a 16-year-old working in a nursing home. It's disheartening to realize that I was already facing moral injury in healthcare at this young age. I came to understand that the nursing home paid low wages to the CNAs and persistently operated with inadequate staffing levels, creating conditions conducive to rushed care that fell short of the standards I would expect for a loved one or myself.

I resigned from my position at the nursing home and secured a job as a unit clerk at the local hospital. This role proved fulfilling. Our modest hometown hospital had a compact emergency department with around six beds and a small inpatient unit of about fifteen beds, typically with only four to eight occupied. As the unit clerk, I handled phone calls, transcribed orders, and prepared necessary paperwork for patient admissions or transfers. Given the hospital's size, doctors or physician assistants (PAs) weren't always on-site. I was responsible for calling them and summarizing why their presence was required. In critical situations, such as a severely ill patient, I played a role in coordinating helicopter services for transport to our facility. In hindsight, it was a considerable responsibility for someone between 17 and 20, but I embraced it. Seated beside the nurses, I gained valuable insights into nursing and medicine. My desk was also strategically positioned across from where doctors and PAs dictated charts, letting me absorb a wealth of knowledge regarding the description of various patient presentations.

As the time for college approached, my primary concern was the financial burden associated with tuition, room, and board. My research indicated that scholarships for medical school were rare, leading me to expect significant student loan debt. Sadly, I closed some doors due to financial concerns. Looking back, I wish I had been more adventurous in applying to out-of-state schools. Financial apprehensions led me to accept the University of Northern Iowa science scholarship. Additionally, the lack of exposure to anyone in my family or their circle attending out-of-state colleges made it challenging to envision an alternative path.

A testament to the generosity of my hometown, I was fortunate to receive enough scholarship funds to cover my first-year room and board. Recognizing that most of these scholarships were one-time awards, I understood that I'd need employment to manage room and board expenses for the subsequent years (two through four), as I was committed to avoiding student loans. This led me to discover the Resident Assistant (RA) program, which appeared promising. The role entailed living in the dorms and helping the residents, primarily maintaining order and providing guidance. RAs were tasked with organizing programming, including educational sessions on topics such as dating, safe sex, the dangers of alcohol, and nutrition. Additionally, we coordinated many social events featuring food and crafts.

Reflecting on my experience as an RA, I now see it as excellent preparation for my current roles as an emergency doctor and facilitator for professional development. As an RA, we underwent basic first aid training and had a first aid kit. I was often the first point of contact for my residents seeking assistance with minor medical issues, from Tylenol[®] and Pepto-Bismol[®] to minor wound care. Occasionally, I had residents who required hospitalization, frequently due to alcohol-related incidents. Discovering someone in the bathroom, covered in a rather alarming, brightly colored emesis—indicative of a mixed fruit punch and alcohol concoction gone awry—if they could not stand, I had to summon an ambulance.

In my role as an RA, having our own rooms was important. Our rooms served as a space where residents would discuss various topics—from relationship dilemmas to contemplating significant changes like switching majors or studying abroad. This experience taught me the art of active listening, connecting residents with on-campus resources, and establishing healthy boundaries. An open door signaled my availability for impromptu conversations, while a closed door communicated that I was resting or studying, and if someone knocked, it had to be important. While I cared deeply for all of my residents, I also was focused on getting into medical school. I protected my study time, including going to the library some nights to ensure no interruptions. I recognized there were always two RAs on call and that I didn't always have to be there.

One of the most significant parts of my time as an RA was forging a deep friendship with Jen. We first met during RA orientation in the spring of our first year and quickly became inseparable. Our bond extended to similar fashion tastes, leading to instances where we would unintentionally show up wearing the same top or sporting matching nail colors. Jen, hailing from Gary, Indiana, with a 78% Black population, had a different perspective from mine, from a small, nearly all-White hometown in Vinton, Iowa, of about 5,000 residents.

Rounds were an essential activity of being an RA.

Several times throughout the night, we'd meet with another RA and walk the building to ensure safety and reasonable order in the dorm. Jen and I took no joy in enforcing some rules, yet we also knew that it was our job to ensure a safe and promote a restful environment late at night. I didn't drink alcohol in high school, and college was the first time I witnessed binge drinking culture up close and the consequences of excessive drinking. Jen and I would much rather wrap up rounds with no incidents to get back to watching one of our shows, getting back to studying, or just back to sleep, as weekend rounds included a post-bar close walk around 3 am.

While we didn't seek it out, we wouldn't ignore, even among the most popular athletic teams, flagrant and excessive drinking that violated the university policies. The first night Jen and I encountered one of these ragers, we were met by very large, very intoxicated football players. We were both sophomores and new RAs. One of the rules about being an RA is that you can't touch the alcohol or really make anyone do anything. Together, Jen and I used a combination of grace and assertive energy to persuade the residents to dump a hundred beers.

The scariest night was when a fire broke out in the dorm. Our staff meeting was interrupted by the fire alarm going off. There had been so many issues with the fire alarms that year, resulting in alarm fatigue among the residents. We were taught that we weren't supposed to knock on doors during a fire. Yet, we all instinctively knew that the alarms had malfunctioned so many times that year we had to knock on doors, as people would assume it was a false alarm, yet again. We began pounding on doors to get everyone out.

Until that point in my life, I never considered myself the person who ran towards a fire. Yet, Tammy and I ran towards the smoke with a fire extinguisher. We found the room, touched the door to see if it was hot, and then opened it, and Tammy blasted the couch with the extinguisher. The fire was extinguished! In case you're wondering, it was started by a resident playing with a lighter and lit a stray string on the couch. Being an RA taught me how to channel courage, from minor interpersonal conflicts to an actual fire. Emergency doctors are often described as the specialty that runs towards chaos and metaphorical fires, and I see much of that courage forged in the halls of Bartlett.

These various roles I took on during my youth not only instilled in me the importance of hard work but also offered valuable lessons in leadership. My hall coordinator, Tammy, emphasized the "assume goodwill" principle in her interactions with dorm residents. This perspective encouraged approaching situations with the assumption that individuals might not be aware of the impact of their actions, fostering a constructive dialogue. The amalgamation of these experiences has undoubtedly contributed to shaping the doctor I am today.

Above all, I am profoundly grateful for the deep and enduring friendship that blossomed between Jen and me. Our ability to seamlessly reconnect, even after weeks of not communicating, speaks to the strength of our bond. It is impossible to be friends with a Black woman in America and not consider the impact that race has on her life and our interactions. Jen didn't have an agenda to educate me about what it was like to be Black. But through the vulnerability of being friends, I got glimpses and sometimes deeper views into what she experienced, and later, her Black husband, Dre, experiences in our country.

The first glimpse came when we were in college, and we were talking about getting pulled over. I had been pulled over one time in my entire life, and it was in my hometown for a good reason. I had never been pulled over in the city where we both went to college. Jen and I had ridden in each other's cars a lot, and Jen had a similar, if not better, driving safety style as me. She shared that she had been pulled over five times during her four years at our college. I had heard about "driving while Black," but hearing it firsthand and seeing its impact on my friend was a deeper level of understanding. I have read many books on the Black American experience. Yet, no amount of reading replaces making relationships and getting to know people and their stories.

Another pivotal moment in the relationship came many years later after George Floyd's murder. I was listening to a podcast, and I appreciated the conversation. I forwarded it to Jen. She replied along the lines of, "Why do you think this is of interest to me?" I had a choice. I could not respond or display the White fragility of "I'm trying to have a dialogue, and you won't engage with me." I did neither. We had a brief call on the phone. While I had many times previously heard the concept of avoiding placing emotional labor on underrepresented groups to engage or educate, I had to sit with that. I had invertedly done it to my best friend.

I didn't go to college seeking a Black friend. I was open to new experiences with people, and along the way, I found Jen. I think it's worth pondering your social network and considering if it is overrepresented with "just like me" people. We all gravitate and connect with people, "just like me." The concept of "just like me" can help you consider many aspects of your social network. Far from a complete list, consider age, geographic background, presence of disability, sexual orientation, and professional, cultural, political, religious, and racial background. As I write this book, I've reflected that my network has skewed heavily toward physicians (a group of people I love). Yet, I've also realized that it has hindered my view and that spending time with a broader array of professionals from tech, law, and creative pursuits has deepened my awareness.

To move beyond "just like me," networks requires vulnerability. Conversations may not start as quickly. There may be a few moments of awkwardness or even navigating a potential trust gap. Yet, we are all people. The ability to connect is universal. Misunderstandings and conflict can happen. I've had some very heated conversations with friends of different political persuasions. In Stephanie Foo's book *What My Bones Know*, she shares this concept of allowing for both the rupture and the repair of relationships. To be human and in relationships with people includes small and large ruptures or conflicts. After reading Foo's book, I realized there were many moments where I let the rupture define the relationship. I didn't make space to allow for the repair, the chance for continued dialogue, and the potential to deepen our relationship.

Going back to the tense moment with Jen, that was a rupture. I had a choice: choose my comfort by ignoring her response or pick up the phone and say, "I missed something here, and I think I hurt you. Can you fill me in?" That's perhaps the easiest part because what comes afterward is taking it in. Do not push it away, but open your heart to hear it.

Reflect:

What are some of the early workplace experiences and relationships that have affected the way you practice today?

_____

_____

_____

_____

Reflect:

Consider your network. Are there opportunities to connect with a broader variety of people?

_____

_____

_____

_____

Reframe:

Consider a rupture (or conflict) with another person; it could be someone from your personal or professional life you no longer speak to or actively avoid. Was there a missed opportunity for repair? Would there be a way to explore reconnecting safely?

_____

_____

_____

_____

Respond:

Based on the reflection and reframe, is there an action you'd like to take regarding your network, or are you seeking an opportunity to invite a repair moment?

_____

_____

_____

_____

Reimagine:

This chapter opened with the power of an early shadowing moment that affected the trajectory of my professional life. Can your workplace provide more opportunities for young people to be exposed to the medical profession? For example, is there a shadowing or volunteer program? Along with benefiting young people, you may find it an enriching and meaning-making endeavor for your staff.

_____

_____

_____

_____

Resources:

Take Our Daughters and Sons to Work Day, learn more about the purpose of this day and when observed:

https://daughtersandsonstowork.org/

How to Be an Antiracist, by Ibram X. Kendi

Legacy: A Black Physician Reckons with Racism in Medicine by Uché Blackstock

Belonging in Healthcare: The Better Allies® Approach to Creating More Inclusive Workplaces by Karen Catlin (also listen to Moving Beyond Performative Allyship: Insights from Karen Catlin, episode 39 of *Heartline* podcast).

The concept of "just like me networks" was introduced to me by Sharee Johnson, psychologist and coach for physicians through the Recalibrate© program. Learn more at www.coachingfordoctors.net.au/

PART 2: THE MESSY MIDDLE

Andrea Austin

CHAPTER 4

BREAKING POINT: NAVIGATING DIVORCE AND SELF-DISCOVERY

"Through an incredibly shitty period of your life, you are allowed to have joy in the middle, beginning, and during whatever part." — Dr. Andrea Austin, on Heartline podcast, Feb 14, 2023

Fifty percent of Americans will get divorced at some point in their lives. This process can be filled with pain, uncertainty, and the unraveling of dreams. My journey through divorce began during medical school, and it made me reflect on the unique challenges that women physicians face regarding relationships, marriage, and the complexities of life while doctoring.

While I'm not a relationship expert, I feel there is much to learn from my experiences trying to partner as a woman becoming a doctor. The time pressures we face and the culture of perfectionism can take a heavy toll on finding and being a good partner. As we start this chapter together, I want to be honest about my shortcomings and the lessons I learned from my divorce.

While my divorce was undeniably painful, there were also moments of unexpected happiness and fun. Despite the turmoil, I was surrounded by supportive friends and engaged in activities that brought me joy. It was a reminder that there is always a flicker of light amidst the darkness. These moments of pleasure were a lifeline, keeping me afloat during the storm. It's a realization that I wish I had remembered during other challenging times, like my deployment or the COVID-19 pandemic.

Now, let me take you back to the beginning of my marriage. I got married at the young age of 22. In hindsight, I realized how little I knew about myself and what I needed from a partner. As a driven undergraduate and medical student, I focused primarily on checking off the boxes of academic success.

Side note: I like to call this the achievement treadmill. Signs that you're on the achievement treadmill are that you look for external sources of validation, frequently feel like you're not in control of how fast or the incline, and you're exhausted. Whether by design or inadvertently, many things in medical education and, later, the medical-industrial complex are incentivized to keep doctors on the achievement treadmill.

Back to 22-year-old Andrea: there was little time for self-reflection and exploration of my desires and aspirations. Marriage, for me, became just another item on the checklist—a natural progression after completing undergrad and entering medical school.

My first husband, Matteo, was a Swiss foreign exchange student whom I met when I was 15 and profoundly affected me. He was introduced by a friend serving as his host family. His olive skin, jet black, thick hair, and soccer player physique were irresistible. He was intoxicatingly handsome, and he had a magnetic pull on me. Our year of dating was intense and filled with new experiences and emotions I had never encountered. However, the foundation of our relationship was built on codependency.

One year into our dating, Matteo fell into a deep depression. Looking back, his depression likely reactivated some of the dynamics around my mother's episode of depression. I knew the depression was not his fault and was a neurochemical imbalance. I felt like our relationship crumbled around that same time, but leaving him felt cold, and I feared I could make his depression worse, even trigger suicide. This led to the development of a codependent dynamic in which I felt like I was responsible for his well-being. I stepped into the caretaker role and out of the girlfriend role. Instead of a give and take, a dynamic of me being the fixer, planner, and problem solver for everything developed. The hyperfunctioning that I honed during my childhood was on overdrive with the struggle to balance being a great girlfriend, working, and studying.

Not only would I be an A student, but I'd also be everything to everyone in the dorm as an RA, and with my free time, I'd be encouraging Matteo. Being mired in everyone else's lives kept me from pursuing self-discovery. Aside from my friend Jen, there wasn't anyone checking in on me. Not that I blame them; my external armor of *"I have it all together"* was ironclad.

I needed more self-exploration and introspection to prepare to be a partner. The academic demands and the necessary volunteering or work experience to get into medical school take up a lot of time. Only later, when I found myself deeper into the relationship, did I realize the magnitude of what I had committed to and the lack of a solid foundation we had built. I also didn't know how to be with Matteo without being codependent.

Codependency is defined as "an emotional and behavioral condition that affects an individual's ability to have a healthy, mutually satisfying relationship.[8] It is also known as "relationship addiction" because people with codependency form or maintain relationships that are one-sided, emotionally destructive and/or abusive." For me, the mutually satisfying part was lacking. Sure, there were some exhilarating moments, especially in the first year and later on trips to Europe, but overall, it was a net negative for me. It was not just a hard season but a slog that I felt required to stick out, likely activated by the depressive episode Matteo experienced early on and relapses throughout our relationship.

Many people, especially women, are drawn to medicine because of its inherent caretaking aspect. We thrive on taking care of others. I encourage aspiring and current doctors to consider whether their caretaking tendencies cross over into codependency in their relationships.

As our marriage began to fall apart, it became increasingly apparent that I had unintentionally enabled a codependency that showed up as me trying to pick up the pieces and shield him from failure. I forgot that while I was an aspiring doctor, I could not heal a person's internal wounds. To have the courage and clarity to leave, I had to confront the damage I inflicted that led to the end of the marriage.

I realize more factors influenced my decisions. Growing up in the Midwest, it was a cultural norm to get married around 22. Many examples from my family and friend group supported this pattern, with couples who had been together since their early twenties and were genuinely happy. For some, this dynamic worked out well. From my observations, the key for these couples is the ability to grow together. No one is the same person years after meeting their partner; life experiences change everyone.

Adding to the complexities, being a woman in medicine

comes with inherent expectations and pressures. We receive overt and subtle messages to be pleasing and accommodating. These societal messages can influence our behavior, and in my case, they played a significant role in my decision to stay in the relationship, even when it got into emotionally and physically abusive cycles.

If you are contemplating a career in medicine, particularly young women, pause and reflect on whether you genuinely have the time and space to get to know yourself. Understanding what you need and want in a partner is vital before starting a lifelong commitment. Building a solid foundation of self-awareness is critical to navigating the complexities of a relationship while pursuing a career in medicine.

The decision to get divorced was both slow and fast. Shortly after getting married at 22, I received an email that was the proverbial straw. We were both supposed to graduate college simultaneously; my husband didn't walk and sat in the audience with my parents at the graduation ceremony. Considering his shy and non-conforming nature, I thought little of it then. However, about a month after our wedding, his father sent me an email containing my ex-husband's college transcript. It revealed that he had failed all the courses in his last semester and had not graduated.

I read the email while surrounded by coworkers at my

summer research job. The shock, surprise, and heartbreak hit me all at once. I recall that young 22-year-old version of myself, excited about starting medical school and working hard as a research assistant. As I absorbed the information, my heart raced and pounded with surprise and profound disappointment. Yet, my colleagues beside me saw no external reaction as we worked that day. I wanted no one to know that something was amiss. This was typical for me in those years; my perfectionism kept me from sharing anything that could dent the image that I didn't have my life together.

This situation shows an unhealthy form of compartmentalization. I stayed at work all day, numb, detached, and brooding over how to react when I got home. Later, I'll discuss strategies to be more aware of when we're compartmentalizing and question if it is necessary or simply more of an avoidance strategy. We'll also discuss how to move through emotions after necessary periods of compartmentalization in a healthier way.

So, after receiving the email that day, when I went home, I stormed through the front door, fueled by anger and disappointment. I couldn't hold back any longer. I had to confront my ex-husband about what I had learned.

I looked him in the eye and said, "I received an email from your father today. I know now that you failed your last semester and didn't graduate. This is not okay, especially since you lied to me."

The air was thick with the ferocity of my words. I demanded answers, desperately seeking an explanation for failing his classes and lying. Then came his response, "It doesn't matter anyway. You're going to be a doctor," he quipped back at me.

In that instant, as his words hung in the air, a realization washed over me. His response was profoundly disappointing, but looking back, it was at least honest. Yet, I wouldn't process the meaning behind his words. Instead, I went into hyperfunctioning overdrive and employed my favorite persona, the fixer. I began brainstorming ways he could go back to college and some work he could do while in school. He was indifferent to my long, wandering list of potential solutions.

The argument began to fade, but not because anything was resolved; it was more the exhaustion of tears and circular conversations, with the knowledge I had to be up in a few hours. As I lay in bed that night, looking up at the ceiling, I knew the marriage was over. My thoughts took on a repetitive, shame-inducing chorus. How could I end a marriage after two months? I thought about all the celebrity couples that get a divorce after a few months and how I had judged them as immature and stupid. Getting a divorce after a few months of marriage didn't seem all that unreasonable. Unfortunate but not unimaginable.

Some may be wondering why it upset me he didn't graduate college. Simply graduating college is not necessarily correlated with intelligence or work ethic. But I was learning what I want and need in a partner. I like to read and talk about politics, culture, and art, and I want to do this with the person I share my life with. I also had many family members struggle with unemployment, limited by their lack of education. While I didn't have complete clarity on my wants and desires, I knew I wanted a partner who shared my intellectual curiosity. I yearned for a partner I could connect with deeply on a philosophical level, something I later called "brain sex" with my now husband. I hoped this intellectual connection would extend long past the more superficial aspects of physical attraction. While plenty of intellectually curious people don't attend college, it was a shorthand for me, especially when I hadn't been exposed to more people with varied life experiences.

In addition, I wanted a partner. What stung so much was that I would be the breadwinner for all of us under every circumstance. I don't mind making more than my partner; I mind when we're not in a partnership. I couldn't articulate it, but in my bones, I knew I needed someone who could take care of himself. Take the lead, plan ahead, and frankly be self-sufficient, as I knew I would work many long hours. I knew I didn't want a grown child. I was outgrowing this codependency phase of my life.

I desired a genuine partnership built on trust, support, and shared values. At that moment, I knew it was time to walk away and seek a future where I could find the love and companionship I longed for. However, I lacked the courage and knowledge to move forward. Our marriage stayed in a suspended state of dysfunction for about another year.

One of my other go-to strategies when life gets hard and I don't know how to proceed is to read books. I also spend time alone, walking, and journaling. Medical school started a few weeks after the disclosure, and the pace of medical school left no space for me to think about how to extract myself from this failed marriage. Nearly every waking thought was focused on studying, and there was a deep uneasiness I wasn't good enough to be there.

I only got into one medical school. I applied to seven schools, a smaller number than many. I was overly concerned about the cost of the applications. Only getting into one school activated an intense level of imposter syndrome, and when medical school began, I was all in. I put my marriage on pause and bottled all my emotions deep down inside me.

It wasn't all bad, either. Becoming a doctor was my dream, and the complexities of the human body and the science behind it genuinely enamored me. Medical school became my refuge, where I found comfort in pursuing knowledge and the companionship of my brilliant classmates. While many people reminisce that their high school or college years were their best, medical school was the best time of my life until that point. Despite the marriage difficulties and suffocating imposter syndrome, I found a real sense of purpose and deep friendships in medical school. Fortunately, there was a summer off between the first and second year, and it involved a few weeks away from Matteo.

For most, the summer between the first and second year of medical school is the last summer break we experience as medical students. Yet, my summer break was interrupted by my military service obligation. Right after my medical school acceptance, I signed up to be in the Navy. I was attracted to the idea of serving my country and, honestly, that they would pay for medical school. Also, I had a deep desire to leave Iowa. While I knew little about the military, I knew there were no Navy bases in Iowa.

So, while most of my classmates went on vacations, I went to Officer Development School in Newport, Rhode Island.

The days were filled with nonstop activity, beginning at the crack of dawn and continuing until late in the evening. Amidst the chaos, surrounded by fellow newly minted Navy officers, I still found an internal quiet and processed the last year and the collapse of my marriage. A quiet strength was growing in me, and I was sure I would figure it out.

I was so ashamed that my marriage was ending. Again, listening to my inner voice, I knew I needed to confide in someone. I had not shared what was going on with any of my friends or my parents. I knew it was a risk to share what was happening, and I felt the safest person was a friend from my medical school class, Miranda.

Miranda was slightly older than the rest of us because she hadn't pursued medical school right after her undergraduate studies. Originally from New York City, her life experiences differed from most of us from Iowa, where most of our med school class originated. I was captivated by her background, her writing pursuits, and the incredible things she had done. She was mature, engaging, and hilarious, too. Being around her, I sensed that she was a safe person to confide in, someone who could understand even if she hadn't experienced a mistake of the same magnitude.

Until this conversation with Miranda, everyone I talked to about my relationship thought it was an incredible fairy tale. Marrying my high school sweetheart, a foreign exchange student, and going on European adventures together—people found it so romantic. Miranda provided a different perspective; she didn't find my story romantic and said divorce was a reasonable option. The validation was like a salve on my soul. I started to feel more whole and like I could trust myself to navigate this situation.

Going through a divorce was undoubtedly challenging, but I found comfort in moments of raw vulnerability with people like Miranda and others who showed tremendous kindness and compassion. My friends from that period saw how broken I was and how much pain I was in, and they loved me anyway. Once it was out that the divorce was happening, we planned a party. As I walked down the hall of our medical school on the night of the party, I saw June, one of my classmates. She looked tired, and although that was not so unusual, I could sense something more profound in her face. I invited her to the divorce party and later learned she was also going through a painful breakup. That year, I learned the power of vulnerability. My friends later told me that in the first year of medical school, I was uptight and not that fun to be around. By removing the veil of perfectionism, I began to make deep friendships and had many fun experiences I still cherish today.

Along with medical school, the Navy played a significant role in helping me channel the fighter inside of me. One of the most memorable experiences of Officer Development School was the USS Buttercup ship simulation. This Navy ship simulator lives indoors, but within minutes of being aboard and traversing the compartments adjoined by watertight doors, it's easy to forget that it's a simulator inside a building. The exercise begins with the ship slowly filling with water. We had to work as a team to save the ship. We patched holes and ran pumps to drain the water. Though safety monitors were present, the experience felt uncomfortably realistic. The water level rose, reaching our necks, and shorter individuals even had to tread water at times.

Through these Navy adventures, I discovered an inner strength I never knew I had. As Glennon Doyle beautifully says, "We can do hard things." Each challenge I faced in the simulations and drills, from jumping off the high diving board into a dark pool, firefighting, or working to save a ship with water up to my neck, revealed the depth of my resilience and capability. I could feel the energy and determination to navigate through the turbulent waters of divorcing while returning to my second year of medical school.

As doctors, our grit can be a strength and a weakness. Grit can keep us in harmful situations. We may fall into the sunk-cost fallacy, in which we are reluctant to let go or abandon something or someone because of how much time we've invested. I had been with Matteo for six years, which weighed on me. How could I let go of a relationship that I had for this long? It is hard to acknowledge that something you've been working on, whether a marriage or a job, is not working. The first step is to stop digging a deeper hole. What helped me let go of this marriage was to step out of my perfectionism. A part of me was worried about what other people would think about the end of my marriage. I finally realized this was my life, my story, and nobody knew the inside of my marriage. It didn't matter what others thought about divorcing a mere year into my marriage. I was suffering and living with toxic codependency. While my ex may have been doing his best, I also knew he couldn't grow into the partner I needed. It wasn't my job to stay and fix him.

As I began rearranging my condo for one, I felt my heart sink. Would I love again? Or was my career the love of my life? A small splinter of clarity began to emerge. I knew I'd be better off alone than in a relationship that didn't light me up for the rest of my days. I boldly chose myself, my career, and my future happiness. I started to hear my inner voice and trust her a little more.

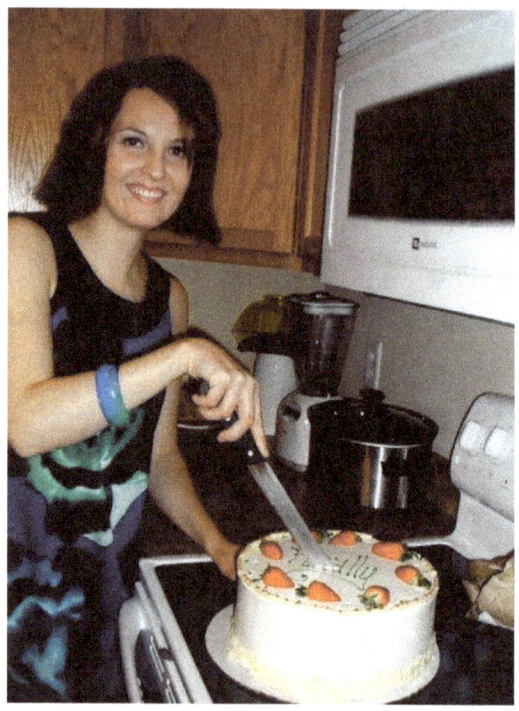

Divorce Party, winter 2009. Cake says, "Finally."

Reflect:

While this chapter focused on romantic relationships, take a broad view of your relationships. Reflect on the quality of connection, honoring of boundaries, and your ability to be authentic with those individuals, whether romantic, friendships, or family members.

_____

_____

_____

_____

Reframe:

Are there any mindset shifts that need to occur to improve the quality of your relationships? For example, do you believe that you are worthy of love?

_____

_____

_____

_____

Respond:

What action must you take to improve your relationship(s)? Maybe it's a difficult conversation that needs to occur.

_____

_____

_____

_____

Reimagine:

How can we change pre-medical and medical education to support healthy relationships for doctors?

_____

Resources:

The book I read in my car and kept hidden under my driver's seat while considering leaving was *Too Good to Leave, Too Bad to Stay* by Mirak Kirshenbaum. I am immensely thankful for this book, which gave me the language to describe my ambivalence and helped me gain the clarity to leave.

The Gottman Institute: using a research-based approach, there are many useful resources, including a full list of their books. www.gottman.com/

Anyone, including doctors, may experience domestic violence. Reach out for help at the National Domestic Violence Hotline. www.thehotline.org/, text 88788, or call 1-800-799-SAFE (7233) in the United States.

CHAPTER 5

THE HIDDEN CURRICULUM OF MED SCHOOL

"We've been taught to not prioritize self-care for so long."— Dr. Jen Wagner on Heartline podcast, Oct 10, 2023

The hidden curriculum of medical school is the untold lessons that shape us beyond the classroom walls. Sharee Johnson, the author of *The Thriving Doctor*, shines a light on this subtext of medical school, in which perfectionism, stoicism, and cutthroat competition perpetuate.

Stoicism ≠ stoicism

Acknowledging the difference between stoicism and Stoicism, the latter associated with Stoic philosophy is essential. It is vexing that they have the same spelling, which must be clarified. My friend and colleague, Dr. Dan Dworkis, author of *The Emergency Mind*, describes beautifully how Stoic philosophy can help navigate the complexities of life and medicine. To be stoic (little s) is defined by the Oxford English Dictionary as "the endurance of hardship without the display of feelings and complaint." Anyone who reads *Meditations* by Marcus Aurelius, a famous Stoic (capital S), knows that he sheds light on life's challenges and, rather than no emotion, he provides tools to cultivate equanimity. When I speak of stoicism in this book, it will be about the hidden curriculum's emphasis on stoicism, the expectation to restrain emotions unrealistically. Stoicism resonates as a powerful tool for many, and I encourage reading *The Emergency Mind* for practical tools to incorporate those strategies into your practice.

Now, let's explore stoicism in medical culture. We're expected to suppress our feelings, even regarding our medical problems. My first rotation in med school was General Surgery, and I started on the thoracic surgery service. On that first day, I rounded in the intensive care unit (ICU), caring for a patient who had just undergone a miraculous lung transplant. I felt awe and appreciation for being trusted to review this patient's chart, followed by a short history and exam. Even the 5 am early rounds couldn't dampen my excitement to be in the clinical environment.

I followed all the infectious disease guidelines carefully, aware of how immunocompromised she was due to the medications required for her body to accept her new lungs. Handwashing, masks, gowns—check, check, check. By 4 PM, after a solid twelve-hour day, our team desperately needed a caffeine boost. We grabbed some coffee to keep the fire burning. A subtle but pressing discomfort was creeping up in my neck and shoulders. I dismissed it as related to my first day with a stethoscope around my neck. I needed to ditch that anyway; surgeons don't wear stethoscopes. With my coffee in hand, I eagerly joined the evening rounds.

The following day, I woke up at the unholy hour of 3 AM, drenched in sweat. Every bone in my body throbbed with pain; my temperature was sky-high at 104 degrees. No amount of denial would change the fact I had the flu. At that moment, a mix of panic and frustration washed over me. *"How am I the one person in Iowa who had the flu in July? Oh, crap! This is terrible! They'll never believe I'm sick! Surgeons are tough, the toughest of the tough, and here I am, a mess on day two of the rotation. I'm done."*

After a few minutes of wallowing in self-pity, my thoughts shifted. *Oh, no! I had rounded on that lung transplant patient just yesterday. Please, please let her be okay.* I silently pleaded to the universe. With a heavy heart, I set my alarm for 4:30 AM, determined to call my chief resident and explain my feverish state. But alas, the fatigue and near delirious state of fever stole my consciousness, and I slept through that blaring alarm. When I finally woke up at 6 AM, feeling even worse than before, panic gripped me like a vice. I had invertedly committed a mortal sin in medicine: I had not shown up. On day two of my surgical rotation. My career was definitely over.

Surprisingly, the chief surgical resident was kind and believed me. I know that seems small, but in our culture of medicine, it is common for people to either not believe you when you're sick or think you're a wimp for not coming in. I shared with him my intense fear I may have transmitted the flu to our lung transplant patient, and he told me not to worry and that he'd keep a close eye on her. To my knowledge, the lung transplant patient did not contract the flu, likely due to me wearing a mask during my morning rounds.

I stayed home for two days, the length of my fever, but on day three, I returned despite a profound fatigue. I felt like I was walking with concrete blocks attached to my shoes. Despite the blanket of fatigue, the work was undeniably fascinating.

The surgeons, from the residents to the attendings, were great teachers, and the operating room was an intense and exciting place. One of my most memorable experiences was assisting (holding a retractor or suctioning) during a case where the surgeons performed a colon interposition for esophageal replacement. This involved removing the esophagus (due to cancer) and replacing it with the colon. The surgeon looked at me and said, "Do you want to perform an appendectomy?" I looked back at him, bewildered. He explained that there was no definitive evidence on whether someone could get appendicitis after the colon was moved into the chest, and he removed the appendix as a precaution. He passed the linear stapler to me, and I fired the cutting stapler to remove the appendix. It was exhilarating!

Yet, the hours were very long, and in my post-flu state, the fatigue was inescapable. I'm usually a two-cups-of-caffeine kind of person. A morning boost and, occasionally, an afternoon pick-me-up if the workload demands it. But during that rotation, in my post-flu state of exhaustion, I consumed four to six caffeinated beverages a day. Without this constant stream of liquid energy, my body threatened to succumb to the merciless clutches of sleep whenever I sat in a lecture or at a computer trying to type notes.

Now, after two weeks of this caffeine-fueled frenzy, a fiery sensation accompanied my trips to the restroom. It was an intense burning during urination. I had never had a urinary tract infection (UTI) before. Like many doctors or soon-to-be doctors, I resorted to the dangerous practice of self-diagnosis. A UTI seemed the obvious answer.

Shortly after arriving at my primary care doctor's office, I provided a sample of my urine, ready for confirmation of my self-diagnosis. The physician assistant walked into the room and casually informed me that my urine appeared normal. I sat there confused. It felt like I was peeing shards of glass. I shared how much pain I was in and pleaded for some explanation. She leaned forward in her chair and, calmly and caringly, said, "Tell me what's been going on in your life."

I recounted the last few weeks of reduced sleep and the

recent flu. She followed with, "How much caffeine have you been using?"

After my sheepish response of 4-6 cups of coffee or soda daily, she replied, "I believe you have chemical cystitis." Medical translation: I had inflamed the delicate lining of my bladder with my excessive caffeine consumption. I had never heard of that, but as a new third-year medical student, I figured that wasn't surprising. My bladder was in such agony I would try anything to find relief.

She prescribed a medication called phenazopyridine, a blissful numbing agent for my inflamed bladder, and gave me some valuable advice—no caffeine for at least a week. The fiery pain dissipated. We usually categorize UTIs as minor complaints- but my adjacent problem gave me a new sense of empathy for how uncomfortable the condition can be.

As the weeks passed, I cautiously tried to reintroduce caffeine into my life. But alas, the consequences were swift and unforgiving. Like clockwork, the sharp pains during urination returned, reminding me that my battle with caffeine-induced cystitis was far from over. As a student of the scientific method, I reasoned that our diagnosis had been confirmed, and the no-caffeine plan had to persist a while longer.

Now, my intention in sharing this story is not to deter

you from indulging in your beloved caffeine (though moderation is always wise) but to shed light on a crucial part of physician well-being. Doctors are human, too. We get sick and injured. We should never feel ashamed for taking time off when we're ill and for the time necessary to recover. Ironically, many of us routinely write sick notes for our patients to miss work, yet we won't ask for a note for ourselves.

Also, the purpose of sharing this slightly embarrassing story is to show the lengths and absurdity we go to keep working despite clear physiological signals of fatigue. I imagine if I had stayed home for another day or two and slept, a therapy I have prescribed hundreds if not thousands of my patients, I would have returned to work slightly tired, but not at a level that required me to chemically burn my bladder with caffeine.

When you are sick or injured, your judgment may be impaired. You might require a fellow physician to step in and say, "You need to go home. We've got it covered. Take care of yourself, and we'll check on you." It may seem like a basic concept, but doctors frequently overlook it. Throughout my training and beyond, I have seen or heard of distressing scenarios that underscore this very point; I'll share a few such stories:

One of my colleagues, Dr. John Love, shared his

experience with a self-diagnosis that has gone awry. After minimizing his symptoms and attributing them to anxiety, he later correctly diagnosed himself with a life-threatening pulmonary embolism.

In another instance, a doctor suffering from a gastrointestinal illness found herself dehydrated and in need of an intravenous drip. Yet, astonishingly, she roamed the hospital halls, attending to patients with an IV pole in tow. This story is a testament to the dysfunctional lengths we will go to fulfill our responsibilities. This story is not rare; in some places, it's viewed as a badge of honor to have seen patients while pushing your own IV pole.

Beyond cruel, just gross is the story of a doctor who faced criticism and shame for calling out sick due to diarrhea. I remember the chief resident's words, laced with callousness, suggesting that a few minutes in the bathroom should not prevent one from seeing patients for the rest of the day.

A colleague confided that during her surgical residency, she was shamed while in active labor. She kept working until she could not stand, and due to the pressure to work until the literal last possible moment, she was forced to sign out her patients between contractions.

Those outside the medical field might be astonished by these stories. Friends who are not in medicine share how they take mental health days when needed. I must confess my intense envy towards them, as I yearn for this rest occasionally. I have found cases throughout my career that have profoundly shaken me to my core. Yet, in our medical culture, there is an unyielding expectation to soldier on. It does not matter if one is mentally, emotionally, or physically exhausted—we push through. How can we ask our colleagues to cover for us when they're tired too?

So, what is the solution? It requires a comprehensive overhaul of the medical culture. One of the most damaging yet well-intentioned constructs that emerged during the pandemic was the portrayal of healthcare professionals as heroes. We are not heroes; we are humans who require sleep, rest, and time for play. Please note these are distinct entities, and we will dig deeper into their significance later in this book.

We urgently need more doctors. Many healthcare teams run understaffed, and some of us have resorted to working fewer shifts than we want, aware that we will face constant pressure to take on more shifts than whatever number we agree to. The current staffing models fail to consider that doctors get sick, become parents, and we experience the sickness or loss of family members, all predictable and valid reasons for time off.

Last, let us revisit the day my body ached before the

fever emerged. Looking back on that day, I recall the profound discomfort in my neck and shoulders. However, I was so detached from my body that I did not recognize the signs of impending illness. Throughout medical school and residency, we are trained to ignore our body's signals. We are taught to power through fatigue, hunger, sleep deprivation, and even illness.

The paradox of our medical education is profound. In honing our diagnostic acumen, we learn to find the slightest signs and symptoms of disease and injury in other people. To do so, the hidden curriculum lures us into believing we must detach from our bodies, even when they are screaming for us to attend to them.

To reclaim our well-being, we must focus on breaking free from this harmful pattern. We must reestablish a profound connection with our bodies, listening to their cues and respecting their needs. We must foster a culture where physicians can acknowledge their vulnerabilities, seek help when necessary, and find support without fear of judgment or stigma. Breaking the cycle begins with each individual, but it is a collective responsibility to reshape the landscape of medicine into one that nurtures the health and humanity of its doctors.

To start this transformation, we must address the challenge of denial. There's a saying that denial is the first symptom of every illness. While we may always gravitate towards denial, we can begin to question it. When the thought of "I'm not sick" arises, pause and ask yourself, "What evidence supports or contradicts this statement?" Additionally, cultivate a low threshold for seeking medical attention. If you cannot schedule an appointment, confide in a trusted colleague and share what you're experiencing. They may offer objective feedback, such as, "You look a little pale. Let me take over your remaining tasks so you can seek medical care."

Embodiment therapy focuses on reconnecting with one's body. Although I have not undergone formal embodiment therapy, I have learned an introductory exercise through my mindfulness practice.

***

Exercise: The Body Scan. Start with your head and work your way down to your toes. Ask yourself, "How does my head feel? Am I experiencing any tension?" Then, scrunch up your face and release it. Repeat this process for your neck, shoulders, arms, etc. Many times, I discover that my neck and shoulders are tense. By engaging in proactive body scans, I can prevent neck pain flare-ups.

Last, in episode 86 of the podcast "*We Can Do Hard Things*," Jen Hatmaker discusses treating your body as a person. Instead of berating myself with thoughts like,

"You're so fat, lazy, and slowing me down," I converse with my body as a friend. I say, *"Hey sister, it seems like you're tired. What can we do? Maybe a short nap?"* Note that I said to nap and not pound excessive amounts of caffeine. Or *"Hey girl, your neck feels pretty tight right now. Let's stretch for a couple of minutes. I've got a yoga class booked for us later this week."*

Some of you may roll your eyes at this concept, but let me ask you this: How is the self-flagellation system working for you? While we can't always protect ourselves from the shame and dysfunction of medicine, we can avoid the second arrow we inflict on ourselves. We deserve to be our best advocates for our emotional and physical health.

Reflect:

As a doctor, you spend considerable time thinking about other people's health. Let's check in on your health:

What is the name of your primary care doctor?

_____

____

When was the last time you saw your primary care doctor?

_____

_____

_____

_____

Describe your overall state of health.

_____

_____

_____

_____

Reflecting on your health, is there a goal you'd like to focus on or improve?

_____

_____

_____

Reframe:

What mindset shift may need to occur to help with your well-being? For example, it may be recognizing dichotomous thinking, such as "I can't be healthy unless I get to x number of pounds." or catastrophizing, "I can't call in sick because then the clinic would fall apart if I wasn't there for a day."

_____

_____

Reimagine:

What would your life look like if you could reach your health goal?

_____

_____

_____

_____

Respond:

What steps do you take to progress toward the health goal you've identified?

_____

____

Resources:

The Emergency Mind book and podcast by Dr. Dan Dworkis, www.emergencymind.com/

Dworkis, D. & **Austin, A**. Being Stoic When it Counts. *From Self to System – Being Well in Emergency Medicine*, www.acep.org/siteassets/sites/acep/media/wellness/acep-from-self-to-system-book.pdf

CHAPTER 6

WOMEN TALKING: BREAKING THE SILENCE OF SEXUAL HARASSMENT IN MEDICINE

"We all have experiences and circumstances in life that come up... We need to change the stigma around that conversation... If in those moments of when they really need something, we listen without judgment." — Dr. Jen Wagner, on Heartline podcast, Oct 10, 2023

Looking back on medical school, I found one lecture jarring. The topic was inappropriate sexual relations with patients. In one study (that relied on self-disclosures; thus, it is undoubtedly undercounted), 2% of physicians reported having sexual relations with at least one patient.[9] The professor closed with, "Don't molest, date, or have sex with your patients."

I sat uncomfortably in my seat, thinking about how much trust I placed in the faculty at my medical school and the aspiring doctors who sat around me. It would be much later in my career that I became more aware of the long history of doctors abusing their patients and colleagues. Disturbingly, there continue to be recent examples of this abuse. Far from a complete list, but a few cases that serve as stark reminders of the sexual violence that doctors have perpetrated:

1. George Tyndall, University of Southern California gynecologist, accused of sex abuse. Hundreds of women reported that Tyndall touched them inappropriately during exams.[10]

2. Darrell W. Harrington, Harbor-UCLA Medical Center director of graduate medical education and a designated institutional official, resigned after two lawsuits alleged that the center ignored complaints about sexual misconduct and discrimination by former orthopedics chief Louis Kwong for years.[11]

3. Larry Nasser, a former physician for American gymnastics, extensive abuse of women and girls.[12]

What strikes me now, looking back on my medical education, is the lack of acknowledgment and strategies to prevent and respond to harassment and assault within our profession. In one study on sexual harassment in medical school, approximately one in three medical students reported sexual harassment by a faculty or staff member. The rate was slightly higher when asked about experiencing harassment by a peer.[13] For me, the problem of sexual violence in medicine starts from within. How can we ask our patients to trust us when we can't even trust our teachers and peers? The problem is rooted in culture, and while microaggressions seem far from the act of rape, there is a continuum of violence. The first step is often othering and dehumanizing women. Thus, a microaggression is not micro at all.

Why does sexual harassment and worse still perpetuate in medicine? Dr. Anitha Menon, in a 2020 essay, asserts that sexual harassment is baked into the culture of medicine. It is a method to exert power and promote the status quo of the patriarchy within the house of medicine. She links sexual harassment to this larger context of gender bias. The lack of proper lactation rooms and protected time to lactate, inadequate family leave, including maternity leave, the decrease in promotion rates, the scarcity of women in senior roles, and the persistent pay gap are all part of a larger social construct that contributes to maintaining the patriarchal structure of medicine.[14]

Looking back on the times that I have been sexually harassed, seeing it through this lens, it would have been so helpful to know that it was less about sex and more about power dynamics. Overlay the military hierarchy on healthcare; it is not surprising that I had these experiences. When thinking about the power dynamics, for me, it helps to think of sexual harassment as akin to bullying, which is all about power over. The sexual component is a fast track to humiliation because it activates the programming that we've received since we were little girls to be demure, and if we are "good girls," we won't attract this behavior. Thus, it is easy to turn inward and blame ourselves for mistreatment when it occurs.

Misogyny is woven into the fabric of our profession. I, like many others, have faced instances of harassment throughout my medical journey. It ranged from subtle comments and demeaning remarks to more overt misconduct. The worst part was the normalization of these behaviors. They were shrugged off as jokes or dismissed as insignificant. Many of these instances occurred before the term gaslighting was mainstream, and looking back, this was another effective tactic to make me question myself. Gaslighting is a form of manipulation in which the abuser sows self-doubt in the victim's mind, which leads to the victim feeling "crazy" and questioning her sanity.

The weight of silence in the face of harassment has affected me significantly. I've questioned whether speaking up would matter. I've also considered the potential fallout on my career. Yet, I'm convinced that collective silence only perpetuates the cycle of abuse and lets perpetrators continue their actions unchecked.

During my intern year, as a lieutenant in the military, I had to wear my khaki uniform under my white coat while on inpatient services. On this day, I was covering for an off-duty fellow intern. She had a complex patient, and my attending instructed me to consult a specialist for his expertise. I went to the specialist's clinic next to the hospital for recommendations.

I knocked on the door and was invited inside. I introduced myself, explaining the challenges we were facing with our patient and our specific questions related to management. The attending physician, seated behind his desk, rolled his chair closer to me and unabashedly fixed his gaze on my chest. I could feel my face turning red as discomfort flooded through me. Shame coursed through my veins, and I began wishing my chest was smaller. Not that he shouldn't be harassing me, but how could I make myself literally and metaphorically smaller to escape this humiliation?

After what felt like an eternity, the specialist concluded the interaction by suggesting, "Why don't you come back to my office tomorrow, and we'll discuss this in more detail." Then, under his breath but still audibly, he added, "I like redheads." I walked as quickly as I could back to the resident workroom.

Sitting at my computer, I had trouble concentrating on my notes. I briefly considered reporting the incident. Yet, I doubted anyone would believe me or take action. I also began rehearsing what I would say and then thought that maybe it wasn't a big deal. Perhaps this was the first time he did something like this or the only time he would do this, and who was I to derail his career? I began blaming myself that the khaki top accentuated my chest and that the incident wouldn't have happened had I only been wearing baggy scrubs or the Navy Working Uniform. I quickly minimized my truth and began to form excuses to protect him. Looking back, it was a near textbook example of how women internalize these aggressions and blame themselves.

The most I could muster was sharing the details with the intern I was covering for, who was another woman. When she returned the next day, I briefed her on the patient's issues and our need for ongoing recommendations from Dr. McCreepy. I didn't go into detail but conveyed that I thought it was an unusual interaction. I recommended she call and not visit his office alone for recommendations the following day when I was scheduled to be off.

When I returned after my day off, I anxiously asked if anything had happened to her. To my relief, she replied, "No, he provided the recommendations, but he did ask where you were." I had successfully avoided Dr. McCreepy, but the nagging thought lingered: How many other women had he subjected to such behavior? Was my experience the worst of it? I feared that it wasn't.

Years later, as an attending physician, I invited several of my closest women attending friends to my home for a movie night featuring "Women Talking." The film portrayed a group of Mennonite women who, through conversation, discovered that they were being drugged and then violently sexually assaulted by men in their community.

As we watched the movie, we paused it many times throughout the night. One of my dearest friends from medical school, who now lived in San Diego, spoke up and said, "Andrea, do you remember that night in Texas? We were at that bar with all your Navy friends, and that guy hit me on my ass really hard."

My heart began pounding, my stomach dropped, and a cold sweat developed on my palms. I felt so ashamed for not standing up for her that night. I remember looking at one of the senior officers who saw what happened, and he shrugged his shoulders and flashed a smile. At that moment, I chose my comfort over standing up for my friend. Frankly, I was worried that if I said something, it would blow back on me. After all, we were at the bar; I knew that was often used against women when they made reports of sexual misconduct. The irony was that I didn't want to be there that night, but I went anyway, hoping it would be a way to break into the boy's club.

I apologized for not standing up for her that night, and she responded with understanding. We all shared our struggles with responding in the moment when faced with such situations. From what we've learned in trauma literature, there are several common responses. While fight and flight receive much attention, we now understand that freezing is a prevalent trauma response as well. Fawning, characterized by being friendly and soothing, is also a response to trauma. Recognizing freezing and fawning as common responses among women when facing harassment and assault helped me forgive myself and others when reflecting on my lack of action that night when my friend was slapped.

Then, another woman in the group spoke up. "Who was it? Who slapped her?" I hesitated for a moment, contemplating whether to reveal his name. Ultimately, feeling safe and trusted by these women, I decided to share it.

"Hmm," she murmured. "He snapped my bra when I was a medical student."

Damn it. This was a pattern. Snapping a bra? It was so juvenile and disrespectful. And she was a vulnerable and impressionable medical student—another example of how humiliation is used as a way to exert power over women.

I won't reveal this man's name in this book. However, I share these stories because women and all individuals must engage in open conversations about this topic. I now regret not reporting or speaking up with a near-equal measure of self-compassion, recognizing the larger societal and cultural context within which these incidents occurred. While not as egregious as some of the sexual misconduct examples at the beginning of this chapter, gender bias and sexual harassment are reported as the top reasons women leave medicine.[15]

Later, during my internship, I presented a patient to a male attending in the emergency department. I was sitting in a rolling chair, talking through the case. He was standing, and then he lifted his leg and propped it up on the desk, like Captain Morgan, with his leg raised high. The position he assumed brought his crotch uncomfortably close to my face while I was sitting in a chair. It was awkward and uncomfortable. I remember gradually wheeling my chair back and leaning away, trying to create some distance between my body and his crotch. He wore this big grin, almost as if he knew exactly what he was doing.

Again, looking back, had I been taught that sexual harassment was more about power dynamics, I could have pulled myself faster out of the initial shame and maybe stood up for myself. Many of us were told that because 50/50 women and men are in medical school, everything is fine, and there is nothing to worry about. Then, we get into these situations, and it causes cognitive dissonance. Part of the strategy must be educating all medical students on the current state of sexual harassment and abuse. So much more must be done to change the culture to ensure it's safe to report, but at least being honest about the prevalence is a starting place.

Years later, I shared this incident with another male attending physician. He responded, "I doubt he understood what he was doing at that moment."

Even if the attending didn't intend to invade my personal space with his crotch (just writing those words speaks volumes for the inappropriateness), I was taken aback by how quickly my male colleague dismissed what had happened. A simple acknowledgment such as, "Wow, that must have been awkward," or other supportive exchange would contribute to feeling more psychologically safe at work.

Fast forward to years later, as an attending physician, during a lull in a shift, a few of us were chatting about the fall of a large corporate management group and the consequence of many of the physicians potentially needing to buy tail coverage. This specific type of malpractice coverage extends past the original policy. Typically, the tail is covered when you leave a position. Unfortunately, the corporate management group declared bankruptcy, which left physicians in the expensive and stressful situation of paying for tail coverage. The male attending began to joke that that's not the kind of tail he wants to go after. Later, during the same shift, when I brought my lunch to my workstation, and he also had his lunch, he said, "Does this make this a lunch date?" My appetite was gone, and I tried to find the appropriate reply that would both shut the conversation down and be pleasing enough to ensure he didn't retaliate.

I call these types of comments casual sexism. They're small comments, passed off as jokes, but they are hurtful and distracting from the important work we're trying to do: care for patients. These comments and the mental gymnastics I must do to create distance, buffer myself, and calculate the potential impact on my career if I push back increase my cognitive load.

Is it any wonder women emergency medicine physicians leave, on average, 12 years earlier than our male counterparts?[16] It is this steady stream of bullshit that disproportionately affects women that contributes to our burnout.

Many times, instances of harassment are subtle. Still, when I reflect on every experience of harassment I have encountered or witnessed, my body instantly feels a shift, signaling that something is wrong. As doctors, we are repeatedly taught to ignore our bodies and suppress our feelings. As women in this society, we face the added pressure to downplay our intuition. When these two aspects collide, it creates a powerful, suppressive force. Now, I have become highly attuned to the sensations of my stomach dropping, jaw tightening, and heart skipping. It doesn't automatically mean something terrible is happening, but I have learned to pay attention to these bodily shifts. I ask myself why I am feeling this way. Is someone behaving inappropriately? Or is it triggering memories of past traumas? Instead of dismissing these signals and assuming I am mistaken, I take the time to pause and examine my emotions.

In the book *Blink* by Malcolm Gladwell, he explores how we can make quick assessments and act before our mind is fully conscious of what or why. We now understand from the trauma literature that our brain is intricately connected to our vagus nerve, which communicates with our internal organs. Our brain may pick up on subtle cues that something is amiss, even if we cannot consciously articulate it. Our brain signals our vagus nerve, triggering a response in our bodies. So, I urge you to listen to your bodies in these moments, for they may be trying to keep you safe. If more of us actively pay attention to these signals, it could be a part of the solution to reducing sexual harassment and worse in medicine and the world.

Harassment in medicine exists on a continuum, ranging from microaggressions to sexual assault. Insults like complaining about a woman taking maternity leave contribute to setting a tone and culture where women are viewed as inconvenient, problematic, and weak. This creates a dynamic that fosters an environment where harassment can thrive and lays the foreground for more egregious acts. It's understandably difficult for the individual to speak up during one of these events. Frequently, a bystander may be witnessing the event as well. We need allies to step in and speak up. Also, we need to normalize and accept that the freeze or fawn response may prevent victims from speaking up in real-time. When they step forward later, we need to understand this may be related to the trauma of the event versus trying to discredit them for reporting later.

I am grateful that many men are committed to this journey and have become excellent allies to me and my colleagues. I highly recommend the books *Athena Rising* and *Good Guys* by Dr. Brad Johnson and Dr. David Smith for practical strategies for men to increase their mentorship, sponsorship, and ally behaviors.

Returning to Dr. Menon's article, she highlights that the quest to irradicate sexual harassment has paradoxically helped perpetuate it. When the stakes are so high that reporting can lead to either party quitting or being fired, we can't get to a place where we can work in psychologically safe places. Part of the path forward involves incorporating the restorative justice practice, which could be a way for people to return to work in some instances. Restorative justice focuses on making amends through reconciliation with the victim and the community.

I can only speak for myself; the harassment I experienced during my career didn't need to end the perpetrator's career necessarily. If there had been a genuine act of owning or acknowledging what happened, it would have made me feel more comfortable. A restorative act, such as working on a committee to improve the workplace for women, would have increased my trust in the system.

Several situations described occurred while I was on active duty. The Veterans Administration (VA) recognizes that sexual harassment is considered military sexual trauma (MST). Along with the long list of potential mental and physical issues that MST can cause, such as anxiety, depression, and panic attacks, it is also recognized to contribute to attrition. The VA considers job dissatisfaction and a desire to leave the military a consequence of MST. This was therapeutic for me, as it helped draw a through line that these early experiences in my career, despite the many positive ones, left an indelible mark and ultimately made me want to leave active duty.

I still work with the military as a civilian. I love serving my country in this capacity. It was essential to remove myself from the active-duty hierarchy. I can assert myself and use my voice more easily in my current roles. I can advocate for people still on active duty and be the safe person they can contact outside the chain of command.

Note: This chapter may have triggered repressed memories or other disturbing thoughts. Please see the mental health resources on page viii of the book or contact the sexual assault hotline below. Please only move forward with the reflective exercises below if you feel ready and safe.

Reflect:

Reflect on any personal experiences or observations related to sexual harassment in the medical field. How have these instances affected you or those around you?

_____

_____

_____

_____

Reimagine:

Imagine a workplace culture where mutual respect and inclusivity prevail. How would this ideal environment contribute to the well-being of healthcare professionals and the quality of patient care?

_____

_____

_____

_____

Respond:

Consider ways to advocate for policy changes or improve reporting mechanisms within your healthcare institutions to address and prevent sexual harassment. How could restorative justice principles be incorporated into your workplace?

_____

_____

_____

_____

Resources:

National Sexual Assault Hotline: 800-656-4673 or chat online at rainn.org

Hawes AM, Gondy K. Sexual Harassment in Medical Education: How We Can Do Better. *J Gen Intern Med.* 2021;36(12):3841-3843. doi:10.1007/s11606-021-06960-w

Athena Rising: How and Why Men Should Mentor Women by Brad Johnson and David Smith.

Good Guys: How Men Can Be Better Allies for Women in the Workplace by Brad Johnson and David Smith.

Athena Rising and *Good Guys* are fantastic reads for everyone in the workplace. I've learned a lot about how to seek supportive male allies, and it has explicit language and concrete actions to increase male allyship in workplaces.

I recommend the book *Sex Matters: How Male-Centric Medicine Endangers Women's Health and What We Can Do About It* by Dr. Alyson J. McGregor. It describes how gender bias impacts patient care and shows how patient care is largely still viewed through the "reference male" perspective. A fundamental tenet of this book is that patients and doctors are inextricably linked. Sexual harassment of colleagues and patients and the issues raised around misdiagnosis in women are all part of a larger societal context of women being viewed as less than. We urgently need to treat patients and colleagues equitably to ensure medicine is a healing and healthy place for all.

Andrea Austin

CHAPTER 7

SQUARE PEG IN THE NAVY

"Part of being a good citizen is bearing witness to the suffering that they had and supporting them to live the best life that they can, knowing that they volunteered, and they went." —Dr. Andrea Austin reflects on her service in the military and caring for Marines with frequent deployments to Iraq and Afghanistan[17]

Recently, a family friend approached me seeking advice on joining the Navy. I responded, "It made me a better person, doctor, and citizen. I'm proud of my service, but let me tell you, it wasn't easy." At first, it may seem peculiar for someone like me to choose to join the Navy. I come from Iowa, where vast fields of corn stretch as far as the eye can see and oceans are nowhere in sight. It all began with my father's enthralling narratives about his military experiences. Those stories had a remarkable ability to make me feel as though military service ran through my veins.

On September 11, 2001, I was driving my purple Ford Escort to school, enjoying the newfound freedom of having a car. As I pulled into the parking lot, the radio announcer's voice filled the car, revealing that a plane had crashed into the World Trade Towers. Like many others, I thought it might be a tragic accident. However, the shocking reality soon unfolded—it was a horrific terrorist attack. Throughout the day, news coverage consumed every classroom. Seeing my teachers, usually so devoted to their subjects, now paralyzed and overcome with grief left me feeling disconcerted.

In the following years, my interest in medicine flourished, and I found myself drawn to stories highlighting emergency doctors and trauma surgeons serving in Afghanistan. If they could handle the demanding field of emergency medicine in such challenging circumstances, they could thrive anywhere. My early childhood experiences also taught me the importance of service, whether through the military or organizations like AmeriCorps. In my last year of undergrad, I received a long-awaited acceptance letter to medical school. The weeks that followed were a flurry of excitement and preparation. I wasted no time contacting a Navy recruiter and soon flew to San Diego to tour a Naval Hospital. The experience solidified my decision, and after returning home, I proudly took my Oath of Office, officially becoming a Commissioned Officer in the Navy.

Throughout medical school, my military involvement was primarily limited to Officer Development School as I pursued my education as a civilian. However, graduation marked a new chapter as I set off for San Diego to begin my residency. In the previous chapter, I shared some of the distressing experiences I faced during residency and my time in the military. However, it is equally important to acknowledge the positive impact of those mentors and sponsors who stood by my side. Just before my last year of residency, my program director sat me down for a conversation that caught me off guard. He asked if I had ever considered taking on the role of a Chief Resident. The suggestion stunned me, as my imposter syndrome ran deep, and I had never dared to envision myself in such a leadership position. Being a Chief Resident turned out to be an extraordinary experience. I leaned into my academic prowess and took on the role of the lead for our residency curriculum. During this pivotal year, I discovered a profound interest in medical simulation, largely thanks to the mentorship and sponsorship of two remarkable male allies. These individuals consistently displayed professionalism and staunch support, always listening to my struggles and pushing me to reach new heights as a doctor, officer, and educator.

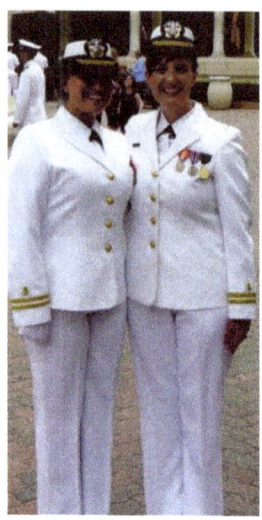

Lieutenant Stein and me on our Navy residency graduation in June 2015.

***

Medical simulation is the creation of real-world situations in the healthcare context. Medical simulation aims to enhance education, assessment, research, and health systems integration, which contribute to improving patient safety and quality healthcare.

At first, my attraction to simulation was more due to my recognition that being an emergency doctor is challenging. We must be ready to care for the young and the old with acute medical and surgical emergencies.

Early in my career, I recognized that I might have to do rare procedures, such as a cricothyrotomy (surgical airway we perform if unable to place a breathing tube the more common way via intubation). Simulation provided a safe way to practice the technical aspects of the skill and the non-technical teamwork, communication, and leadership components of caring for patients.

Later, I became drawn to the psychological component of simulation. Following a simulation scenario, the simulation facilitator leads the team in a debrief. Through debriefing, the team processes the emotional and cognitive aspects of the case. A skilled debriefer can create an atmosphere of psychological safety, defined as the ability for someone to take an interpersonal risk. For example, they verbalized that they were unsure what medication to give or how to proceed at a branch point in a resuscitation.

Debriefs provide an opportunity to reflect and consider the purpose and impact of our work. As odd as it sounds, while doctors do very profound work, we don't have many avenues for talking about the effects of breaking bad news, like a cancer diagnosis, on a patient. The simulations of these cases also enhance the emotional processing capacity that translates into the actual clinical arena.

While I'm still very much drawn to the patient safety and quality implications of simulation, as my career has progressed, I'm more drawn to its ability to contribute to the self-actualization and well-being of clinicians. Simulation lets doctors practice procedures and clinical reasoning, which helps them be more prepared in the clinical environment. Simulation goes beyond the individual; it transforms teams and helps with organizational learning.

Medical simulations use a combination of very sophisticated manikins that can talk, breathe, and other realistic physiologic indicators, along with task trainers that allow for practicing procedures. In addition, standardized patients and participants are trained actors to provide more realism, especially when practicing more of the communication aspects of doctoring. Increasingly, there are virtual and augmented reality options as well. There is even a specialized form of makeup for manikins or standardized participants called moulage, which adds a layer of realism to scenarios.

Along with the psychological component of simulation, I love being creative. Each simulation is like a small play that involves the script, set, and cast of characters, which all combine to create a realistic medical scenario that challenges a group of medical professionals.

I didn't know about simulation when I entered medical school. I wouldn't keep practicing medicine without simulation. Now, when a case doesn't go as well as it could have, I can step back and see the systems issues contributing to a less-than-ideal outcome. I can then go back to the simulation lab or bring the simulation into the clinical space to help a team practice, experiment, and uncover new ways of working together and overcoming systems issues. The ability to bridge work as imagined and work as done and interweave the humanity of healthcare energizes me as a simulation educator.

***

In the Navy, it is rare for residency program graduates to remain as faculty. Typically, you are expected to move to a new command in a different city or even a different country. However, due to my specialization in simulation, I received orders to stay in San Diego and join the faculty—a dream come true. I could continue living in the city I loved while teaching and serving my country.

About six months after residency, I learned I would deploy to Iraq. My reaction was mixed. On the one hand, it was why I joined the military—to use my skills as an emergency doctor and resuscitate patients in austere environments. I craved the challenge that this deployment would bring. But I was overwhelmed at being away from my loved ones for months. I also felt like I had barely caught my breath after residency, and while the deployment was something I wanted to do, it also felt like a massive disruption to life right when I was feeling some normalcy.

Military service inevitably changes you. I remember standing in the coffee line as a fresh intern alongside wounded warriors. It shifts your perspective when you encounter individuals younger than yourself, Marines in their early twenties with multiple amputations, and people for whom I started ketamine infusions to alleviate the unrelenting pain from their phantom limbs when they arrived at the emergency department.

Less than 1% of people in this country have deployed to Iraq or Afghanistan. Many Marines I cared for had been on four or more deployments. These deployments may be as long as a year (rarely even longer), which doesn't even include the pre-deployment workups and post-deployment periods, which frequently keep them away from home. For these brave individuals, four deployments meant about four years away from their families and friends. I can promise no one deploys that frequently for that long and returns without physical and emotional wounds.

Many people will assert that we're a volunteer military, and that's what we signed up for. One of the most hurtful things people could say to me before I left for deployment was, "We're still in Iraq?" The cost of having an all-volunteer military is that we, as a country, have forgotten what shared sacrifice means.

32-year-old Andrea, preparing to deploy to Iraq in 2016, was not nearly as fearless or clueless as the 22-year-old version that had signed up to be in the military. A seven-month deployment presented a disruption to my marriage, life, and career that was daunting. The scariest part was the complete lack of control I had. There was no option to resign or ask to come home- I was along for a ride. A ride that could be extended. A ride that involved being in a combat zone.

***

As the C130 landed in Iraq, I felt slightly better. The back-and-forth regarding whether I'd deploy, when I'd go, to what location, and for how long, including in the days leading to my departure, contributed to my anxiety. As my boots hit the sand, a relief settled in. The clock to coming home had begun.

For the first couple of months, I was in Iraq. While the work was challenging, it was meaningful. We took care of trauma patients, primarily Iraqi soldiers, who had been injured by improvised explosive devices (IEDs) and gunshot wounds sustained fighting ISIS (Islamic State of Iraq and Syria). I began to settle into a rhythm and made friendships with the trauma surgeons and one of the British doctors.

After two months, we were notified that they would replace our team with a medical team from the Czech Republic. This meant we'd be going to Kuwait. Once in Kuwait, we'd be working primarily in a clinic. It was so strange; I went from being scared to be in Iraq to enjoying our work and now disappointed that our team was moving to Kuwait. While safer and certainly better food, it felt like a weird letdown.

When my team arrived in Kuwait, we reintegrated with our original team from California. Yet, a strange divide occurred, and I had no work to do besides covering the clinic one day per week and taking a call night every two weeks. On average, I had about 10-12 hours of work to do a week, leaving excessive downtime.

At first, I thought this was fantastic. After morning muster, I'd return to my room, read, and work on papers or academic pursuits. As an academic physician pre-deployment, I had a stack of projects I had been excited to dig into. By afternoon, I'd go to the gym for one hour. I learned I would get too hungry if I worked out for over an hour. This would mean I'd need to eat more, and the food would not be enjoyable.

The nights were the hard part. I'd watch movies and read books. Occasionally, I'd go to a social activity, but for the most part, I stayed in my room. Leaving my room involved putting on my uniform and boots. The boots. I hated them. They were so heavy, and despite my best efforts to find insoles that would make them more comfortable and the claims by so many people they were comfortable, they weren't for me.

My story is not that unusual. I later learned that many women veterans have permanent foot issues related to footwear that hasn't been designed for women. One of my friends shared a story in which she was issued the wrong size of shoes at a military academy, and her feet sloshed all year. She was told they didn't make boots small enough to fit her feet.

I've spent a long time on the boots issue, but this is a giant metaphor for how we receive real messages that we're not meant to be in the military. Every step we took was a painful reminder. This also extends to more significant issues, such as body armor. Ill-fitting body armor could prevent it from protecting vital organs. It can also increase strain on the neck or other areas, resulting in chronic musculoskeletal issues.

***

Unlike in Iraq, I had my own room. Alone, my mind would sometimes turn dark. One night, my mind seemed caught in a loop. Looking back, it was severe anxiety that, as a Type A control freak, I had usually managed by seeming to exert control over my life. Now, in this room, looking up at the ceiling in Kuwait, I began to spin out. What happens if this deployment keeps getting extended? What happens if we invade Syria? What is the meaning of life? What is the point of this suffering I'm experiencing?

I thought about the M9 in my room and that my ready access to a weapon could quickly end my suffering. I could still think logically and recognized this was a destructive thought and likely a temporary low point. As an emergency doctor, I have spoken with countless suicidal patients and many psychiatrists in consultation to help patients with mental health emergencies. I knew that suicides are frequently impulsive actions, and it is a dangerous combination to have impulsivity, depressed mood, and ready access to a firearm.

I looked over to the "wall of happy," which was every card someone had sent me while I was deployed. My logical, and now my emotional brain, told me it would be okay. Many people loved me, and many people on this wall had deployed and come home, too. While it seemed far off, I hoped to be home again someday.

I knew in my heart I was having a bad night and that all I needed was the gun removed from the room. I wanted it checked back in the armory. Yet, I feared being sent home if I alerted anyone to my thoughts. This would result in being labeled a loser and weak and may end my military career. Worse, it would mean that another one of my colleagues would get activated and yanked from their life to fill my spot.

The military has huge cultural issues that impact mental health. First is the bravado culture, that we are tough and that mental health issues are associated with personal failure. In addition, toxic workplaces in which harassment, bullying, unfair demands, and lack of inclusion exacerbate the likelihood that people will experience mental health events.

I've also noticed that the well-intentioned focus on mental health has led to a one-size-fits-all approach that lacks nuance. For example, I suspect I was experiencing an adjustment disorder, defined as a temporary failure to cope adaptively to a stressful situation. Adjustment disorders are treatable and very common in the military. Adjustment disorders frequently respond well to increased support; most people can return to full duty. Yet, many commanders are reticent to have anyone on their team that could be a "liability." They don't want any potential risk, so they will have a low threshold to send someone home. Ironically, this all-or-nothing approach leads to people suffering in silence and not coming forward for the help that would get them back to being healthy and contributing team members, increasing the risk these commanders are trying to avoid with an all-or-nothing approach.

It seems odd that my mental health was worse when I arrived in Kuwait. It was safer, with more cushier surroundings. Looking back, I fell into the trap of overidentifying with my professional identity. Until this point, my identity was wrapped around being an emergency doctor. Lack of meaningful work, when your identity is tied to work, was a risk to my mental health I didn't understand.

The all-encompassing way we train doctors, with 80-hour work weeks during residency, dramatically contributes to this identity problem. With 12-14 hour working days, it is understandable that people have difficulty developing relationships and hobbies that contribute to a more well-rounded identity.

Along with the issues around identity and self-worth, a lot of my distress was related to a thought error called future tripping. Future tripping occurs when we think about what may happen, which, for many of us, especially when anxious or depressed, turns to worse-case scenarios. Future tripping and negativity bias, in which we focus on the negative, create a powerful thought vortex that can be challenging to escape. Yet, simply knowing these terms can be a powerful antidote.

Sharing my experience of grappling with suicidal thoughts is not easy. Still, being candid and vulnerable about the struggles many face in medical and military professions is essential. We hide behind a facade of strength, fearing the consequences of revealing our innermost thoughts. We downplay our pain, afraid of future overreactions and repercussions.

The next day, I recognized the gravity of the thoughts that had consumed me the previous night. Concerned for my well-being, I sought help from a psychologist attached to the Air Force. Instead of openly discussing my suicidal thoughts, I used the coded language of being stressed and a bit down. The psychologist was helpful, and even though I kept the actual depth of my struggle hidden, his words and guidance provided enough of a lifeline that I felt I could keep going.

Looking back on that night, I know that I was close to falling permanently into the abyss of nihilism. Several years later, when attending a lecture by Dr. Amanda Dinsmore, she shared a helpful framework. Suddenly, my brush with suicide made so much more sense. It deeply troubled me for years, mainly because I didn't understand the thought fallacy and how to prevent it. She shared a diagram that her team, The Whole Physicians, created about future and present detriment, inspired by the book *Happier* by Dr. Tal Ben-Shahar. I've further adapted the diagram to mirror some of the language from earlier in the book, including the achievement treadmill.

The key to fulfillment is staying present. When we

overly focus on the future, we often get stuck on the achievement treadmill rather than enjoying what we have now. We can also fall into the trap of worrying about the future and that nothing will get better, and that gives way to nihilism. This lack of hope can show up as learned helplessness behaviors and contribute to a depressed mood. Conversely, suppose we lack hope for the future. In that case, we can focus on "getting mine now," which leads to hedonistic behaviors. We need to cultivate presence and agency to craft a fulfilling life.

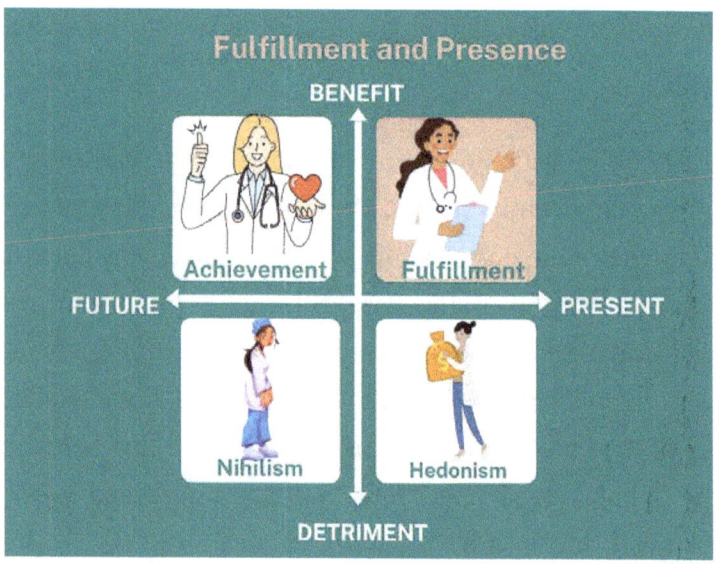

Image credit: Dr. Andrea Austin made with Canva. Image adapted from Dinsmore, Amanda MD; Cazier, Laura MD; Morrison, Kendra DO. Wellness 911: You've Arrived: Why Aren't You Happier? Emergency Medicine News 44(4): p 30, April 2022.

Physicians, as intelligent as we may be, are not immune

to the overwhelming burden of mental health challenges. Physicians have one of the highest rates of suicide of any profession. Male doctors have a suicide rate 40% higher than the general population. Women doctors have a 130% higher suicide rate.[18] Every year, we lose hundreds of physicians to suicide, and these numbers may only scratch the surface of the true extent of the crisis. The shame and stigma surrounding mental health leads to underreporting and the misclassification of deaths. It boggles my mind that we don't communicate this risk to people entering medical school and remind them about it throughout their careers.

Similar to military personnel worried about the impact on their careers, physicians also worry about the potential consequences of seeking mental health care. While improving, there are still states that ask invasive questions about whether physicians have ever sought mental health support, even marriage counseling. If disclosed, some states may delay medical licensure pending a review of private and sensitive mental health records or add more evaluations for medical licensure.

While I am an ardent patient safety advocate, the issue with these laws is that they make patients less safe. We need to normalize that most people will seek support. Aside from just living, which involves potential divorce, death of loved ones, and other tragedies that are hard to cope with alone, being a doctor or veteran has its share of challenges. I hope we get to a day when it is more surprising someone hasn't sought the support of a therapist, including in stressful professions like healthcare and the military.

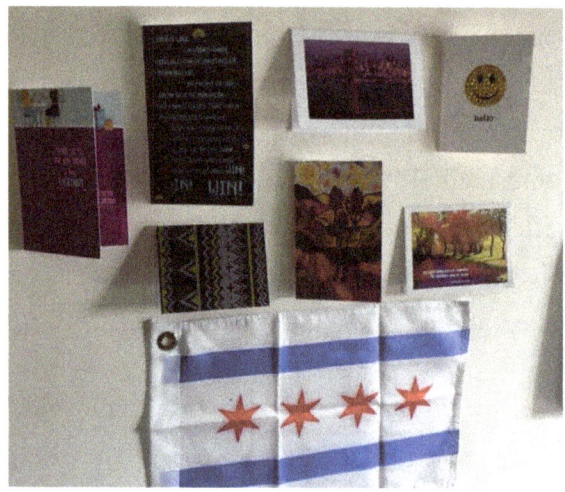

Wall of Happy: Cards and a Chicago flag were sent to me, and I hung them in my room once I got to Kuwait. These cards and gifts saved my life.

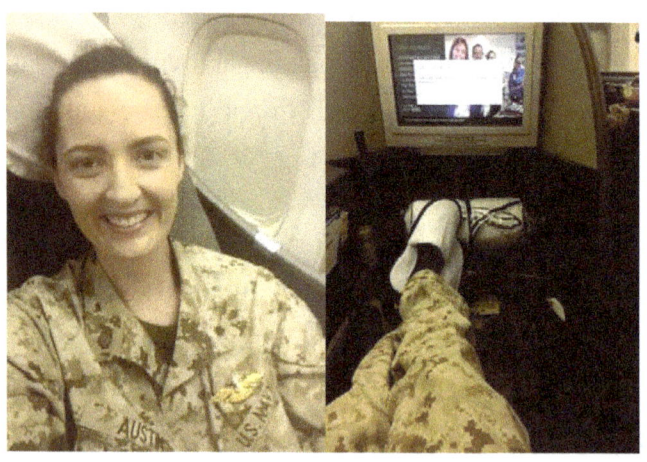

Flight home after 7-month deployment.

Reflect:

How do you relate to your professional identity as a doctor? What are other important roles you have in your life?

_____

_____

_____

_____

Reimagine:

What areas of your life would you like to explore to expand your identity? Consider various relationships, hobbies, or other interests.

_____

_____

_____

_____

Respond:

What's one action you can take to expand your identity beyond being a doctor?

_____

_____

_____

_____

Mental Health Resources:

- Help is available for anyone in crisis, including thoughts of suicide, by calling 988 in the United States.
- If you're a veteran, you may call 988 and press 1 for veteran-specific help. You may also text 838255.
- From the National Alliance on Mental Illness, healthcare worker-specific resources: www.nami.org/Your-Journey/Frontline-Professionals/Health-Care-Professionals
  - To learn more about the crisis of physician suicide and what can be done to help, watch the documentary Do No Harm, www.donoharmfilm.com

Resources:

To learn more about medical simulation, I recommend the SSH (Society for Simulation in Healthcare), www.ssih.org, and Simulation as a Career Path blog at andreaaustinmd.com

Acknowledgement:

I want to acknowledge Dr. Taryn Rose, an orthopedic surgeon who founded a luxury shoe company that uses technology to create custom, comfortable shoes. At the September 2023 Women in Medicine Summit, Dr. Rose measured my feet and noted that my right foot is a whole size larger in width than my left, and this explained the foot pain I had throughout my military career. I hope Dr. Rose's technology will be widely adopted to make comfortable shoes for everyone, especially in the military and healthcare. Shop her collection www.enricocuini.com/.

CHAPTER 8

LaLa Land

"I did probably have enough in the tank to be able to resurrect again and reshift and change. But my heart and my soul had already moved. They had actually called enough." — Dr. Michelle Woolhouse, on Heartline podcast, Aug 22, 2023

Coming home from deployment, a strong desire to leave the military consumed me. The weight of a four-year contract with the Navy called "payback" for their support during my medical school years loomed over me. My orders after residency had initially been for a three-year tour in San Diego. I still owed one more year…and unfortunately, I fell into a predicament of either taking a new set of two-year orders or accepting a one-year billet overseas and unaccompanied, which meant without my husband. Still reeling from the isolation I experienced on deployment, I knew that unaccompanied orders were not something I would entertain.

While considering accepting a new set of orders, I also began to ponder what that would mean for any hopes of starting a family with Chris. Before I married Chris, the topic of having children had come up. Growing up in the Midwest, married couples were expected to start a family. Looking back, I can't recall a single couple from my childhood who didn't have children. So naturally, I assumed that I would want to have kids as well. When Chris's mom asked me if I wanted children, I met her gaze and confidently replied, "Yes." At that time, I genuinely wanted to start a family in my twenties.

I met Chris during my final year of medical school, and we married in my second year of residency. A few women had children in my residency, but their experiences varied greatly. While some faculty and co-residents were supportive and understanding, others were not. More than once, I heard the phrase uttered, "If the Navy meant for you to have kids, they'd issue one in your seabag." It was a reminder that the military expected its members to prioritize their duty above all else, including starting a family.

As military emergency physicians, deployment held immense significance. It symbolized strength and service, offering opportunities to earn a warfare device that would be displayed on our uniforms. People scrutinized our uniforms, assessing the presence of a warfare device and the number and type of ribbons to determine if we had deployed and where we had served.

The idea of deployment activated all those people-pleasing and achievement tendencies within me. I made a conscious decision that getting pregnant before deploying was too risky. It seemed safer to wait until after I had fulfilled my deployment duties so no one could accuse me of "dodging" my responsibilities.

After returning from deployment, my desire to have children evaporated into thin air. Many people have questioned my decision, responding with well-meaning comments like, "No, you haven't missed your window! You're still young!" Some even offer unsolicited advice on fertility treatments and other methods to help me conceive.

When I say I missed my window, I'm not referring to being infertile or entering menopause. It's not a matter of physical capability. Instead, I missed the window of having the genuine desire and capacity to be a mother. The desire to be a mom is essential to navigating the challenges and sacrifices that come with motherhood. The capacity refers to the mental and physical ability to carry a pregnancy and care for a child.

After returning from deployment, I felt mentally and physically drained. The thought of experiencing the physical discomforts of pregnancy, delivering a baby, and then the responsibility of caring for a newborn overwhelmed me. I was struggling to take care of myself, and deep down, I knew I needed to prioritize my well-being. I genuinely believed that if I were to get pregnant, the likelihood of experiencing postpartum depression or worse would be alarmingly high. My emotional tank was running empty, and I intuitively knew that bringing a child into the mix would not be a healthy decision for me.

Over time, I have made peace with my choice of not having children. Instead, I find joy and fulfillment as a supporter and nurturer of my adult friends. Our home has become a sanctuary where friends seek refuge during life transitions, moves, or after heartbreaks. We lovingly call it the "adult rehabilitation and relaxation zone." It brings us great satisfaction to provide emotional support and care for the important people in our lives, knowing we can make a meaningful difference for them.

I've realized that mothering takes many forms and doesn't always involve giving birth to a child. Nurturing and supporting others can be just as rewarding and fulfilling. I've embraced this alternative path, cherishing the deep connections I've built with those around me.

***

As I grappled with the predicament of my orders, it became increasingly clear that I would need to fulfill my service obligation at a new duty station. Guantanamo Bay was quickly ruled out. Going there alone for a year seemed like a recipe for disaster, as I feared the potential downward spiral of isolation. However, another option caught my attention—the Navy Trauma Training Center (NTTC) at LA County + USC.

NTTC was renowned for providing comprehensive trauma training to Navy healthcare professionals, equipping them with the latest advancements in trauma care before deployment. Their training program combined didactics, simulations, and clinical shifts in trauma units to enhance our skills. What intrigued me even more was that the emergency physician at NTTC served as the simulation director—a perfect fit for my educational niche. Additionally, LA County + USC boasted an esteemed emergency medicine program with an all-star faculty.

However, there was one significant hurdle: LA County and USC were in Los Angeles, while our house and Chris's job were in San Diego. It was a considerable distance, raising the question: Could we live apart together?

We discovered that we were not alone in our decision. About 3.9 million married Americans aged 18 and over live apart from their spouses.[19] Each couple has its unique reasons, but in the healthcare field, many of us choose to live apart together (LAT), at least temporarily, for professional reasons such as training, sabbaticals, or accepting a compelling new position. For some, LAT is a temporary arrangement that lasts only a few months or a year, while for others, it may become semi-permanent or even permanent. LAT can also serve as a trial period to assess a new job before uprooting one's partner or family.

After a year of living apart, I gained valuable insights about myself and my marriage. I learned to create clear boundaries between work and home life, something I struggled with before. Instead of working during our limited time together, I focused only on cherishing those moments. This shift resulted in a sense of dating and brought back a deep appreciation for our time together. Technology was an essential tool in maintaining our connection. We eagerly looked forward to our near-daily video chats, and texting provided a convenient way to stay connected throughout the day. However, we valued our independence and didn't rely on constant texts to feel connected.

Living apart was a journey of growth and self-discovery. During residency, I had become reliant on my husband's exceptional cooking skills and stopped cooking for myself. However, during my time in LA, I experimented with cooking and found joy and relaxation in preparing my meals. It has become a form of self-care and a way to express my creativity in the kitchen. I've realized that I can find fulfillment and independence in nurturing myself.

In addition to cooking, I learned to be more self-reliant and focus on my personal security. A scare in my parking garage served as a wake-up call, reminding me of the importance of accountability for my safety. Instead of always turning to my husband for solutions, I have embraced a sense of empowerment and taken on challenges outside my comfort zone. From troubleshooting technology glitches to assembling furniture, I discovered a newfound satisfaction in completing tasks independently. I learned that while we are undoubtedly stronger together, I can stand on my own two feet.

Occasionally, I faced pointed questions and curiosity about our LAT arrangement. Some people found it difficult to understand why we made this choice. For me, part of the decision has involved letting go of societal expectations that dictate a woman must sacrifice her career ambitions. Fortunately, I have a partner like Chris, who supports and encourages my professional aspirations. I have also learned to release the need to explain or justify our decisions to others. Ultimately, it was about what worked for us as a couple at that particular life stage.

My clinical shifts at LA County + USC were a whirlwind of fascinating and challenging experiences. During those two years, I encountered some of my career's most unique and complex cases. I performed and oversaw rare and high-stakes procedures, such as lateral canthotomy, thoracotomy, and cricothyrotomies. The trauma that came through those doors was unimaginable—gunshot wounds, stabbings, and devastating motor vehicle accidents. It was a constant reminder of the fragility of life and the resilience of the human spirit. But it wasn't just about the clinical aspect of my work. It was also about the opportunity to train and mentor hundreds of physicians, medics, and nurses. Many medics I worked with needed more direct patient care experience, and I had the privilege of guiding them through their first CPR attempts and helping them care for dying patients. Drawing from my background as a simulation educator, I introduced a valuable practice into our shifts at LA County—debriefing.

Debriefing is a process where we reflect on our experiences and identify areas for growth and improvement. In simulation training, debriefs have been effective in enhancing learning. So, I incorporated debriefs into our clinical shifts. I would gather the Navy team away from the busy floor to debrief our most challenging cases. And if time didn't allow for an immediate debrief, we had one before going home.

What I saw during these debriefs was genuinely remarkable. The team members opened up, shared their vulnerabilities, and grew closer. They spoke about their discomfort in performing new skills and their uncertainty during critical moments of the cases. They expressed how the patients affected them emotionally and voiced their need for support. These debriefs let them construct deeper meaning from their experiences and find solace in a safe and supportive environment.

Debriefs should be integral to our healthcare practices

as we strive to transform the industry. They provide an outlet for our emotions, helping us process our intense and overwhelming experiences. Debriefs also clarify misunderstandings, identify improvement areas, and facilitate quality improvement initiatives.

A change in the city resulted in letting go of more emotional baggage. Staying at the same program where I had been a resident meant I never truly felt like a respected peer among the faculty. A few less supportive and evolved faculty members took pleasure in reminding me of past mistakes and inadequacies that dated back to residency and refused to acknowledge my growth and transition from resident to peer.

However, changing jobs presented a chance for reinvention. Joining the LA County + USC team, I found a fresh start and a renewed sense of purpose. The Navy doctors had built a solid reputation with the faculty and residents at LA County, and my deployment experience and trauma expertise were highly respected. Instantly, I felt a sense of credibility and could let go of the insecurities that had plagued me as a resident. The leadership at LA County embraced my passion for supporting women in medicine, and I was given the opportunity to reinvigorate the women in medicine group. They appreciated the professional development initiatives I led for both faculty and residents.

What stood out to me the most was the support I

received from the Chair at LA County. He took the time to meet with me multiple times, offering guidance and assistance with my career progression. With his help, I obtained a faculty appointment at USC, further solidifying my standing in academic medicine. When the time came for me to transition out of the military, the Chair even contacted the program I wanted to work at next, advocating for me and speaking to my abilities. The Vice Chairs also played an important role in my journey, generously offering their mentorship and sponsorship. They took the time to meet with me, discuss research ideas, and provide valuable career advice. Their support and belief in my potential gave me the confidence to navigate this pivotal transition in my life. I realized that leaving the military was not a sign of failure but an opportunity for growth and new possibilities. I embraced my true capabilities as a physician and educator.

In some ways, I wish the years in LA would be stretched indefinitely. The experience at LA County + USC was transformative, and the professional growth I experienced was invaluable. However, deep down, I knew LA was not the place I could call home. The city felt too vast, and its energy didn't align with mine. But San Diego beckoned me with its familiar charm and the promise of a place where I could belong.

In the fall of 2019, I resigned from the Navy and pursued an academic position in San Diego. I resigned and eagerly began transitioning to this next chapter of my life. Everything seemed to align perfectly, and I even received a job offer for the position I had interviewed for. I was ready to start a new adventure.

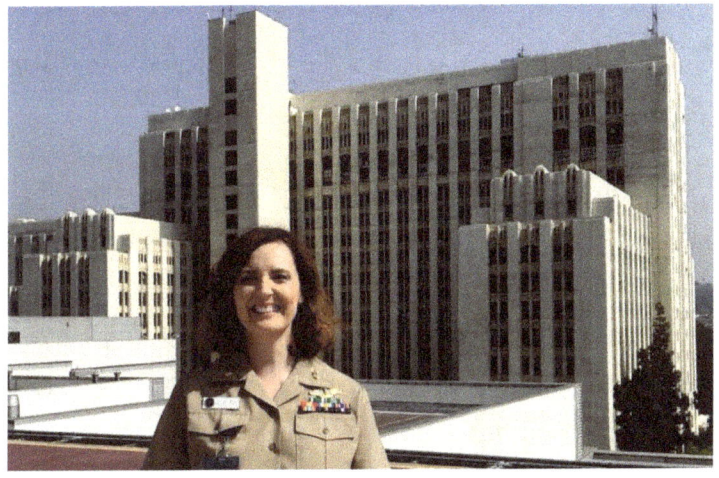

This is my first day as the emergency doctor and simulation director at the Navy Trauma Training Center (NTTC) at LA General, formerly LA County + USC, in front of the old hospital that housed NTTC.

Reflect:

Limiting beliefs are thoughts or states of mind that stop you from doing certain things. In this chapter, I discussed several limiting beliefs. For example, I couldn't work in a city away from my husband and have a healthy marriage. Consider a firmly held belief affecting your joy or fulfillment in medicine right now. For example, "I could never leave my current position; the salary is too good."

Potential   limiting   belief:

_____

One strategy for debunking a limiting belief is examining the evidence. Start with the question:

Is   the   belief   factually   true?

_____

If you're human, you probably wrote yes. Try again. Examine the evidence to determine if it is true. Also, consider if you're unsure and need more information to determine the validity. For example, in the initial example with the salary, do you know for a fact that there are no higher-paid positions available?

_____

_____

_____

_____

Another strategy is, even if it is true, is there any other way to reframe it? For example, the salary may be the highest, but if this job affects your well-being, you may not be able to do it as long as a job that is more compatible with your well-being; therefore, you may not make as much money as if you shifted into a lower-paying, more sustainable position. Or is there a better position for your well-being that pays the same or is even higher?

_____

_____

_____

_____

Reimagine:

Is there a new way of looking at the thought you've attached to the limiting belief?

_____

_____

_____

_____

Respond:

With this new outlook, is there an action you'd like to take?

_____

_____

_____

_____

Acknowledgement:

Portions of this chapter were inspired by the blog post originally published as Living Apart Together by Dr. Andrea Austin.   Nov   27,   2019.

https://feminem.org/2019/11/27/living-apart-together/.
Thank you to Dr. Dara Kass for founding Feminem and Dr. Jenny Beck-Esmay for your leadership at Feminem. Creating a space where we could share stories, get published, and develop connections to navigate the joys and challenges of practicing medicine has been invaluable.

CHAPTER 9

THE PANDI

(As No One Calls It, But My Husband)

"I think both of us have been through a period of probably personal evolution... I think that's important before you think about how you actually are going to support and lead a team because you can't actually do that work if you're not able to support yourself." — Dr. Cheryl Martin on Heartline podcast, January 30, 2024

I want to skip this chapter, yet while painful, the pandemic is a powerful force that led me to revitalize my life and career. I was sitting on my couch at home with my husband on that fateful day, March 19, 2020, when the lockdown order was issued for California. The air felt heavy with dread, and a sinking feeling settled in. As the analogies between COVID-19 and wartime abounded, I began to sense that this would again be a time of stress. Unlike deployment, we didn't know how long the pandemic would last.

Early on, I came across a news story about a young doctor in China in his twenties who had succumbed to COVID-19. His youth was jarring. He was younger than me, and his death forced me to consider my mortality. It was strange, but before I started my deployment to Iraq, losing my life there seemed implausible. It might sound peculiar, but I hadn't known any doctors who had lost their lives in Iraq or Afghanistan. While required to complete a will before leaving, even that didn't make death feel possible.

Yet, as soon as I set foot on that C130 and landed in Iraq, the reality of potential death felt nearer. This feeling would ebb and flow, intensifying during certain moments, like when the wailing sound of an air raid siren pierced through the air while crouched under a table or sitting through a safety briefing about terrorist threats to our base.

As a doctor, one knows there is always an infectious disease risk. From HIV to Ebola, various diseases emerge, and we figure out strategies that keep us safe. The lack of clarity around how COVID-19 was transmitted made me feel like every patient was a potential infectious bomb, and simply, the act of speaking could be the contagious shrapnel that could take me out.

Early in the pandemic, I recorded a podcast with my colleague, Dr. Dan Dworkis, where we dug into strategies for managing the challenges brought by COVID-19. Among them was the advice to confront the worst-case scenario, including the possibility of death. In the first few weeks of the pandemic, I had candid conversations with my husband about my wishes if I became critically ill or died.

The first phase of the pandemic was scary. Yet, the

initial public outpouring of support for healthcare workers, combined with the flurry of activity to keep connected online for information, kept me distracted. As reports poured in from Italy and New York City, I experienced dread mingled with a determination to brace for the inevitable surge.

The start of the pandemic was eerie. The number of patient visits dwindled dramatically in those first few weeks. In one telemedicine shift, I pleaded with the parents of a child who had been in a severe bicycle accident. He seemed drowsy, and my medical instincts told me it could be a severe concussion or even a potential brain bleed. It took all my persuasive skills to convince them that, despite their fears of COVID-19 exposure, an emergency visit was necessary. The pandemic introduced a new layer of complexity to medical decision-making.

The situation was rife with challenges that made it both terrifying and horrendous for healthcare workers. Early on, the scarcity of personal protective equipment (PPE) shattered our trust in the system. Healthcare professionals choose this path to serve, aware of the risks of treating contagious diseases. However, that service comes with an implicit understanding that adequate PPE will be available. This discrepancy between expectations and reality was one of the most disheartening aspects of those early days.

Yet, the stark isolation was perhaps the most soul-wrenching among the hardships. As doctors, forging connections with our patients is fundamental to the therapeutic process. We frequently can't cure or fix; a compassionate word or a reassuring touch is the needed solace we provide. However, as the virus's transmission mechanisms remained unclear, minimizing contact and time in patients' rooms became a survival strategy. When we eventually had access to PPE, wearing it for extended periods became an ordeal. It was paradoxical – the gear we yearned for to ensure our safety at the pandemic's start had transformed into a source of discomfort and exhaustion.

Along with patients, even our colleagues emerged as potential sources of exposure. The once communal spaces like the break room or the doctor's lounge, where shared meals and heartfelt conversations were a balm for our spirits, now stood as high-risk zones to be cautiously sidestepped. The staff was sizable at an ER where I worked, and it used to be routine to enjoy a break with a colleague, sharing food and companionship. But now, our breaks were timed to ensure solitary consumption. The warmth of friendship had shifted into a wariness of potential infection.

In my eyes, the most challenging facet of the pandemic was the unsettling politicization of masks and vaccines. I distinctly remember a patient in respiratory failure, struggling for breath, who muttered, "I don't have COVID," just before I had to intubate him. The following day, I checked on him and received the grim news—he was COVID-positive with massive blood clots in his lungs. He passed away later that same day.

Fueled by the Thanksgiving gatherings, the wave that hit in early December of 2020 was one of my lowest points. Many patients I saw had mild symptoms. It was frustrating to be exposed to the virus while treating patients who might have had nothing more than fever and body aches, especially when they were young and otherwise healthy. The risk of contracting COVID-19 just before the vaccine's availability felt even more exacerbating.

Then came a hopeful time after the vaccines were finally administered. The vaccines proved highly effective, and a sense of security arrived. Even when entering COVID-19 patient rooms, I felt a newfound confidence. This gave way to the disappointment many of us experienced with yet another wave in the summer of 2021, with the rise of the delta variant. While the vaccines offered substantial protection against severe illness, they didn't guarantee immunity from contracting COVID-19. This resurgence of uncertainty and frustration became an unexpected challenge yet again.

By the spring of 2021, burnout engulfed me like never before. I had what some might call a "dream" job in a prominent academic medical center. But the pandemic had sown seeds of doubt about my chosen path. The experience made me question whether I was cut out for this profession. I needed a break, a chance to step away, recalibrate, and explore something different.

Reflecting on the COVID-19 pandemic, I found it exceptionally challenging because it unfolded in waves. Though I had a feeling that it might persist for several years, like the swine flu pandemic, it was still mentally taxing to see these waves crash upon us, seemingly without an end in sight.

In January 2022, I contracted COVID despite being vaccinated. Though the course was relatively mild, it was emotionally draining, and having the virus inside me that had caused such widespread suffering and agony among those I had treated felt like a defeat. It brought back all the memories of the saddest and scariest moments of the pandemic.

The winter surge of 2022 brought with it an unprecedented level of exhaustion among the healthcare staff. This collective burnout profoundly affected how some of my colleagues coped with their frustration, and unfortunately, it manifested in ways that deeply concerned me. One particular aspect that troubled me was the reluctance to allow families at the bedside.

In some hospitals I worked at, policies were still in place that restricted family members from being present unless the patient was in imminent danger of passing away. Once, we treated a patient whose daughter had been by her side throughout her illness, who had COVID. On this specific day, the patient was in the dying process but not at the point of imminent death. Despite that, she was still conscious and able to communicate. My earnest wish was for her daughter to have a chance to spend precious moments with her while she was still coherent and responsive.

However, I faced resistance from a nurse who maintained that family members should be allowed only when death was imminent. I tried to reason with her, explaining that waiting until the last moments meant denying them the chance to connect and share words before it was too late. The daughter had been exposed, and considering that we were all vaccinated and following safety protocols, I couldn't fathom the reasoning behind not letting her be there.

I firmly believed that if we were all vaccinated and taking proper precautions, letting families be present in the hospital was not only reasonable but essential. I emphasized to families that if they were coming in, they needed to adhere to wearing masks and wearing them correctly. As time went on, denying family members and visitors access to the hospital began to feel cruel, and I could see the impact it was having on our patients.

One night, I encountered an elderly gentleman with

chronic lung disease who had a notably low oxygen level. Complicating matters, he was also grappling with dementia. As we prepared to admit him, his daughter was barred from going upstairs with him, as per the hospital's restrictions. This separation caused him immense distress during the journey to his room upstairs. He adamantly refused to be admitted without his daughter's presence.

He was brought back to the emergency room, left off monitors, and without oxygen support. Discovering him in this state left me astonished and concerned. I quickly sought a nurse to understand why he was not receiving proper care. The response was crushing – he was considered for discharge against medical advice because he expressed his desire to leave due to the absence of his daughter. This elderly, confused man, scared by his daughter's sudden absence, was left vulnerable.

Later, I learned that the distress I felt while advocating for this patient was a form of moral injury. I knew what he needed, and getting the system to provide compassionate care was daunting. As the demands mounted and the burnout reached unprecedented levels in these later stages of the pandemic, I saw a distressing erosion of humanity among some healthcare workers. At times, the system seemed to falter under the weight of the relentless challenges. Looking back, it's clear that our response needed a more strategic, sustainable approach. The pandemic was not a sprint but a marathon of endurance, and our staffing models should have reflected that reality.

A more thoughtful approach could have made a significant difference. Rotation strategies could have been implemented to allow frontline workers to catch their breath. For example, ICU nurses could switch to different units like clinics or post-anesthesia care units for a period. This variation in responsibilities might have helped alleviate the overwhelming burden that came with the constant barrage of COVID-19 care.

As I pondered potential solutions, the concept of flexibility needed to be integrated. Offering different avenues within the healthcare sector seemed promising. For example, incorporating telemedicine into the rotation could have provided a welcome change for emergency physicians. These other options would keep healthcare workers engaged in their field but offer a much-needed respite from the frontlines.

The military is well aware of the importance of rest cycles. Navy staff cycle between shore duty and sea duty, understanding that after long stints away at sea and under stress, periods of shore duty are designed to allow for some recovery time. We didn't build in recovery time or the potential for varied work for our frontline healthcare workers.

I would not choose the pandemic. Yet, the growth it spurred inside me is profound, and I know I'm not the same person I would have been without it. I remember being at a yoga class in 2021, and a familiar anxiety crept in when we were instructed to take deep inhales and exhales. My mind rushed to the air potentially full of COVID-19, and my familiar hyper-vigilance began to counteract any calming measures the yoga was meant to have.

I took a child's pose. With my face against the mat, I let out a few tears. I wouldn't be the same person as before COVID-19, but I also felt a quiet hope that I would one day hear people breathing without thinking about COVID-19. I didn't know how or when that would happen. I just sat on my mat, hoping it would happen someday.

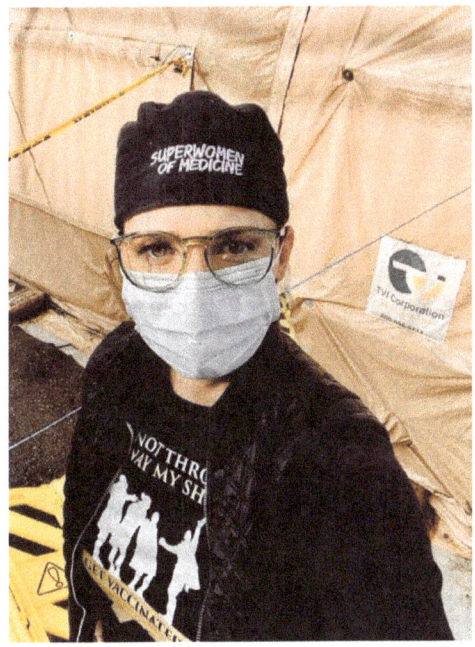

March 2021, vaccinated and tired.

Reflect:

Are any triggers left over from the pandemic that no longer serve you today? Consider avoiding social gatherings, anger towards those who don't wear masks or get vaccinated, and anything that results in a flash of anger, sadness, or other negative emotions that impact your ability to enjoy life or your career.

_____

_____

_____

Reimagine:

The trigger may always be there, yet your response to the trigger may diminish or change. Is there any reframe regarding the story associated with the trigger that you can tell yourself? For example, I had to remind myself that while the air in the yoga studio may contain COVID-19, I was vaccinated, and proven treatments could decrease the severity of the disease and risk for long COVID-19.

_____

_____

_____

_____

Respond:

What action would you like to take to address a potential trigger left over from the pandemic? Please note that this action may involve contacting a therapist, as the cognitive approach of a reframe does not always sufficiently rewire the neurological pathway that has become fast-tracked. We'll discuss this in the next section.

_____

_____

_____

PART 3: THE REVITALIZATION

"Could you accept the burnout? Could you accept that you're having it and that to get through it, maybe look into what you need and what would get you on the path of integrity to practicing medicine in a way that would actually feel good and... in a way that you could show up as your best self?" —Dr. Andrea Austin on Heartline podcast, Mar 12, 2024

While I had experienced episodes of burnout before, the episode that occurred at the end of the pandemic was different. Prior episodes felt temporary, and with a few tweaks, I could bounce back. This one was on a soul level and was a clear inflection point in my life. There's no experiencing life or thinking in the old way; I was changed. During past episodes of burnout, I turned outward. I looked for a solution that would work for someone else and tried it on me. This time, I felt a pull to go inward. After several months, I began to feel a clarity emerge, and an optimism began to surface.

Inflection point + Inner work + Clarity = Revitalization

Revitalization is defined as "imbuing something with new life and vitality." What I like most about revitalization is the "re," emphasizing the past. The past is still there; no matter how painful, it is integral to the revitalization process.

Simply going through something terrible or traumatic will not guarantee revitalization. Many people go through traumatic experiences, get stuck in a trauma loop, and aren't able to move forward. Or they move forward without gaining the insights, and the next time a new trauma occurs, it's like they're going through it for the first time again.

What does doing the work look like? I was once asked how long it takes to recover from burnout or moral injury. I can't answer that question. I can share tools that helped me, and I trust that each physician knows their life best and will take what is helpful and craft their revitalization.

Doing the work, this phrase refers to the life-long process of taking intentional steps towards self-improvement. I want to provide definitions and discuss how different forms of assistance are available to help you do the work or even figure out what doing the work would mean for you.

As healthcare professionals, we refer patients to mental health services, but we don't receive extensive training about the various types of therapy or counseling available. My friend and colleague, Anna Rainville, a Licensed Marriage and Family Therapist (LMFT) and founder of Grounded Roots Mental Health Therapy, specializes in trauma. She categorizes therapeutic approaches into two major types. The first is "top-down therapy," which includes cognitive behavioral therapy (CBT), a specific talk therapy. Psychodynamic and interpersonal therapy are other examples of talk therapy.

The second type is "bottom-up therapy," which utilizes modalities that use body sensations to process memories stored in the nervous system to promote long-term healing. EMDR is an example of this approach. Understanding these options is essential for those seeking a therapist and those providing referrals. Talk therapy has become embedded in American pop culture and featured in countless movies, podcasts, and TV shows. In contrast, bottom-up modalities like EMDR, somatic experiences such as yoga or dance-based therapy, and art-based approaches are just starting to gain more attention. Despite being viewed as "woo-woo," the evidence supporting bottom-up approaches is growing, and large healthcare systems, including the Veterans Administration, are increasingly reimbursing and encouraging these modalities. If you or someone you know has been trying talk-based therapy and not improving, especially if trauma is involved, it may be time for a bottom-up approach.

I also talk about coaching. The International Coaching Federation defines coaching as partnering with clients in a thought-provoking and creative process that inspires them to maximize their personal and professional potential. Coaching is future-focused, meaning there isn't much looking back at the past. While coaching can be therapeutic, *it is not therapy*. Coaches don't treat or diagnose mental health disorders. Coaching assumes that the client can fully manage their own life, and through the partnering aspect of coaching, the client can unlock solutions to be more fulfilled and address life challenges.

Do you need a coach or a therapist? This can be a difficult question to unravel. When in doubt, I'd recommend starting with a therapist. The rate of PTSD in healthcare workers[20] is about 40%, and about 30% of healthcare workers[21] meet diagnostic criteria for clinical depression. Given the rates of mental health conditions, if you have any concerns or others have expressed concerns to you, I highly recommend contacting a therapist.

In addition, as my therapist so brashly stated, we all walk around with our bags of shit. I have yet to meet the person with the perfect childhood, from parenting to schooling to friendships. No one escapes life; some experiences can lead to maladaptive coping mechanisms. While you may meet no diagnostic criteria in the DSM-5, that isn't the bar we're trying to reach. We're talking about thriving, not simply the absence of illness.

Sadly, if you don't choose to do the work, hospitals and state medical boards refer physicians to extraordinarily punitive programs rooted in a culture of shame. I highly recommend reading *If I Betray These Words* by Wendy Dean and Simon Talbot. They highlight the story of a physician on call nearly every day and night who was maligned by his organization and eventually referred to a Physician Health Program. The way he was treated in an intensive residential program was cruel. He ultimately committed suicide. I encourage physicians to reach out for help well before any state medical board or formal actions from employers get involved. Once an outside entity is involved, it takes away the autonomy of the medical professional to choose the approach they prefer and, at a time and financial cost, they are comfortable with.

Addiction also occurs among doctors, and this can vary from substances such as alcohol or opioids. In addition, shopping, gambling, and even internet usage can become an addiction or have addictive behavioral patterns. Addiction therapy is beyond this book. I acknowledge it because it is a real problem, and doctors face a unique stigma compounded by the ease of access to controlled substances.

Even if it doesn't progress to an addiction that meets clinical criteria, many of us spend money in a way to offset the emotional pain of doctoring. I know many miserable doctors. Returning to the Dr. Tal Ben-Shahar framework, this is living in the hedonism quadrant. It's fun to live in; I have designer shoes, purses, and first-class memories to prove it. If those items are within your budget and fulfilling, go for it. There was a phase in which I consumed uncomfortably as a "reward" or "treat" because I worked hard. I deserve it, or on bad days, my job is terrible, and I deserve these fancy things.

In the book *Your Money or Your Life: 9 Steps to Transforming Your Relationship with Money and Achieving Independence* by Vicki Robin and Joe Dominguez, they share that however much money you make, you have to subtract the money you spend to survive doing it. For example, if you hate your job and need to take quarterly all-inclusive vacations to keep yourself going back, you need to subtract those vacations from your salary. I am not against travel. I love it, and later in this book, I'll talk about therapeutic travel, a more embodied way to travel that doesn't have the hedonistic or escape edge that some travel has when we're miserable in a job. When done in line with your values, boundaries, and priorities (including finances), travel is a great way to continue growing as an adult, enrich neuroplasticity, and connect with people.

As I continued my personal and professional revitalization, I didn't feel the need to make huge designer purchases or constantly travel. I found myself more embodied and okay with staying home with less stuff (knowing I already have a beautiful and very comfortable home).

Let's return to the question: coach or therapist? For me, it's both. Different times in my life have required more support from a therapist or a coach. The most important thing is to find coaches and therapists who are well-trained and experienced and keep your interest at heart. For example, in a session with my coach, I kept returning to an encounter with a bully. She stopped me, asked permission to give advice, and then recommended I bring up this past trauma with my therapist.

As I made strides with my therapist and discussed how ongoing support looked, she agreed that a group coaching program for physicians would be a great source of ongoing development. It would be a way to continue to do the work. For me, I still check in regularly with my therapist, as we've determined, at least for now. I work in a high-stress job with ongoing exposure to trauma, and at least monthly sessions are good for me. It helps to have one place to go and be assured that what I share is confidential, and I can cry and process the complex parts of life and doctoring.

Coaching is particularly beneficial when you feel you need to change and are unsure what you want or need. Maybe you're feeling bored or otherwise unfulfilled by a job. Or change gets thrust on you. Perhaps you're being tagged with a new project or running into an interpersonal or team challenge that is new or particularly difficult. My friend Dr. Amy Vertrees introduced me to the term "lifequakes."

Lifequakes come in many shapes and sizes and include the death of a loved one, loss of a job, divorce, or a health issue.

In the current world, and especially in healthcare, we are living through a time of VUCA: Volatility, uncertainty, complexity, and ambiguity. Healthcare is undergoing horizontal and vertical integration, which means the entity you work for may be acquired. It can also mean that doctors are caught between various competing interests. For example, you may face competing interests between patient safety and hospital politics to avoid causing conflict and maintain a contract that keeps your group afloat. The pandemic was VUCA on steroids. The mis and disinformation that followed were, and still is, equivalent to, "Hold my beer," how can we make his pandemic even more awful?

How do we navigate the VUCA-ness of it all? We do the work. One afternoon, I called up a doctor friend and shared a vexing moment on shift. I shared that instead of stifling what I thought, which, after years of doing that, had caused me to nearly leave medicine, I vocalized my concern. I had a difficult conversation with two colleagues about how I felt after an earlier interaction in our shift. To this day, I have a good relationship with both colleagues, mainly due to those conversations. I lamented that I didn't handle the situation perfectly when talking to my friend. My voice may quiver, and I don't always deliver the message in the most

Zen way possible. She laughed and said, "That's what they mean by doing the work." No one said that doing the work is comfortable or easy (note I am a process perfectionist, discussed more in the chapter on adaptive perfectionism). Even though I got through the hard conversation, I will get tripped up by how it unfolded wasn't "perfect." Hard conversations aren't meant to be perfect; that's why they're hard.

Also, while there's a place for emotional regulation, there's a place for emotion. The goal is not to remove emotion from these moments. It's to convey it in a way that doesn't dampen the message. Reflecting on the hard conversation, I know that my colleagues and I relate better because they saw that what happened hurt me. I showed emotion, which was vulnerable. In this vulnerability, we found a connection. The ability to get vulnerable at that moment was built on years of work, and my ability to access vulnerability was primarily based on Dr. Brené Brown's books and podcasts.

Cautionary note: beware of predatory coaching programs. Coaching is still an unregulated industry. There are accreditation bodies, including the International Coaching Federation (ICF), mentioned earlier, with a heavy emphasis on ethical practice. Many times, people contact coaches when they're at rock bottom. While I believe in the value of coaching, don't let it erode your financial well-being.[22]

Read on to craft your revitalization.

Reflect:

What areas would you like to grow more personally or professionally?

_____

_____

_____

_____

Reimagine:

What would support look like to grow in the ways that you desire?

_____

_____

_____

_____

Respond:

What action can you take to start the process of more support on your journey?

_____

Resources:

Dr. Lorna Breen's death inspired me to be vulnerable and share my story in this book. She committed suicide during the early portion of the pandemic. Her suicide was in part due to her fear that her mental health condition would be reported to a medical board or credentialing committee and could derail her career. I saw myself in Dr. Breen and knew that I could have succumbed to suicide, primarily due to the stigma of reaching out for help.

I am a proud ambassador of the Dr. Lorna Breen Heroes' Foundation (https://drlornabreen.org/). Check out their Take Action page for organizational and individual resources, including the toolkit to remove intrusive questions from licensure and credentialing applications: https://drlornabreen.org/take-action/. Consider becoming an ambassador. Encourage your organization to join ALL IN: Caring for Caregivers, https://drlornabreen.org/caring-for-caregivers/.

Andrea Austin

CHAPTER 10

OPERATION HEAL THYSELF

"I was in this cocoon kind of way, and I knew I had to get out. I just knew it on a soul level. I still needed to keep going... reconnect to my heart and find my essence again." — Dr. Michelle Woolhouse describing "breaking" from burnout and her recovery on Heartline podcast, Aug 22, 2023

As the pandemic eased, I thought I would feel better. Yet, as March 2021 began, I didn't feel the renewal in the air. I felt crumpled, crushed, and depleted on a soul level. Early in the pandemic, we went through this honeymoon phase in which consultants, the other doctors in the hospital we call to admit or help with procedures, were kind to us. We were the frontline "heroes." That faded a few months into the pandemic, and the usual antics resumed. It was more challenging because the usual salve of cracking jokes wasn't the same with a mask on, and the occasional hug was unavailable.

The admitting team may resist admissions for various reasons, including concerns regarding compensation for themselves or the hospital. In the ED, we call this blocking. During this pivotal month, when my burnout was at the highest levels, an interaction with a consultant got my attention. I was taking care of a patient with chest pain. He had many risk factors and a particularly concerning electrocardiogram (EKG). I called to admit him, and the physician began with super aggressive blocking. Ultimately, I admitted the patient, but it was hard-fought and energy-depleting. Even the half-apology the consultant offered after interviewing the patient, reviewing the EKG, and agreeing that admission was necessary provided no relief.

As I began to drive home that night, I had pain in my chest. I was 36 years old. I thought to myself, *I'm reasonably sure I'm not having a heart attack. Yet, if I was older, I might check myself into an ER if I was having this pain.* I knew on an intellectual level it wasn't a heart attack. I also knew that something was happening to my body. The emotional pain I was experiencing was affecting me physically.

Looking back, my heart was breaking. Not literally, although there is a medical condition that is, effectively, a broken heart. Takotsubo cardiomyopathy is a type of heart failure that occurs after extreme emotional distress. For example, it may occur after someone experiences a profound loss, like the death of a loved one. The patient will present with the classic signs of heart failure, and testing will reveal a heart swollen from weakening in the cardiac muscle. Takotsubo is the word for a Japanese pot that traps octopuses.

I did not have Takotsubo cardiomyopathy. Yet, I

realized at that moment that all diseases start somewhere. The pain I felt in my chest was not a heart attack tonight. Yet, I could feel the stress on a visceral level, which was not something I could ignore. I knew on a soul level, more powerful and correct than my medical training, that if I didn't find a new way, I would die, literally or metaphorically.

I also recognized that no amount of self-care would get me out of this situation. I was the queen of self-care. I had a beautiful bathtub with various calming aromatherapy concoctions, monthly massages, getting my nails done, getting enough sleep, and exercising. I was doing all the self-care, and I was still miserable on my clinical shifts. I began recognizing the problem—I was happy sitting on the couch with my dogs. I was also pretty Zen floating in the pool.

"It's not always perfect, but my bad days are very tolerable, and my great days are really wonderful." -Dr. Rip Patel, the Heartline podcast, episode 46

My bad days weren't tolerable, and my body's signals were no longer ignorable. Living for the day off would not cut it.

Chris and I took a vacation in the spring of 2021. While mostly resting, I began to lay the groundwork to leave my job. I shared with a few friends I was burned out. Looking back, burnout was the term I used, but it doesn't encapsulate what was happening. Burnout was the only word I had to describe it. Years later, I had the privilege of virtually meeting Wendy Dean, author of *If I Betray These Words*. She said that when she sees burnout, she suspects there is a moral injury at the root. She is a psychiatrist, well-versed in the intricacies of the mind. She posited that almost all physicians that go into medicine are compassionate. It is our nature to help and care for people, and we get an intrinsic reward. Thus, to become burned out usually means that the system has failed both the doctor and the patient. Our burnout is partly rooted in the feeling that we're not caring for patients in line with our ethics or the same way we'd expect a loved one to be cared for.

Moral injury was first coined to describe soldiers' experiences in combat. It refers to the feeling of violating one's conscience or moral compass when one participates in, witnesses, or fails to prevent an act that disobeys one's morals, values, or personal principles. Now, many of us in medicine, primarily caused by the corporatization of medicine, feel we cannot care for our patients in a way that aligns with the ideals and expectations of our medical training.

While I said I was burned out, I had an epiphany after hearing Dr. Dean speak. At the root of the burnout was moral injury. During the pandemic, so many harrowing experiences, on top of the status quo of our dysfunctional healthcare system, caused extreme moral injury.

As we age, we learn more about who we are. I recognize that I am an empath. As an empath, I feel people's emotions profoundly. The emergency department is the pressure cooker of humanity at baseline. Patients arrive at the emergency department bruised, broken, ill, or dying. The pandemic caused extreme distress. Everyone's heightened state during these years was undeniable. Then, add on staffing shortages and all the other barriers that emerged during the pandemic to providing ethical care—it hurt my soul.

I could feel in my bones that I couldn't practice medicine in a way that aligned with my values. I couldn't figure out whether it was this particular place or the specialty of emergency medicine. The only way I could begin to untangle it was to stop. I needed a break. I also needed *to break*. I needed to fully experience all of the heartbreak of the pandemic, deployment, and practicing medicine in a dysfunctional system. I took a 3-month sabbatical to hold space for the breaking and the hope that I would begin to come back together on the other side.

On top of everything else that was dysfunctional about the first year of the pandemic, I worked a disproportionate number of night shifts. Humans are meant to sleep at night, and emergency departments must be staffed at night. This presents a profound problem. While I usually got the recommended hours of sleep or at least caught up after a string of nights, fatigue began weighing on me. It was a deceptive form of fatigue, and I didn't know how severe it was until I got my rest.

"Sleep is a human right." —Dr. Sheri Dewan on the Heartline podcast, episode 40

I'm not going to belabor that sleep is fundamental. There have been so many books written on the topic. If that's not enough, sleep deprivation is used as a torture technique. Also, people forced to stay awake eventually experience hallucinations and psychosis. Sleep is fundamental. I knew this. As I crafted my recovery, I started with sleep as the non-negotiable, aka a boundary I would protect vigorously. All the sleep research shows that going to bed at the same time and waking up at the same time is best. Thus, I found work that would support that goal.

Thankfully, my strong network, built while I was in the Navy, buoyed me during this untethered phase of my career. A friend and colleague forwarded a job opening for an online simulation teaching position—the job posting required six years of simulation experience, which I had met. I reminded myself that the research shows that women won't apply for a job unless they meet and exceed the requirements. I couldn't do that this time; it was time to leap.

I landed the online simulation education position, which was only a fraction of my usual salary. It was intermittent work, which meant this position would cover my sabbatical time…but then I'd need to figure something else out. I knew I couldn't move to the next thing without the sleep and time to rest, play, and regain my sense of purpose. Importantly, this position also allowed for a regular schedule. I began going to bed and waking up around the same time. I believe this was crucial to my healing, as sleep is integral to processing trauma.

One night, with a non-medical friend, I recounted the story of a patient who died from blunt-force trauma to her chest. She was driving down the road when another car crossed the median, crashing into her car, and the force ruptured her heart. How do I know? I saw her heart. We did a thoracotomy, and I saw the ruptured wall of her ventricle. An inoperable injury. It is profound, that moment when you see someone young, and if we only saw her face, she looked serene, different from the catastrophe within her chest. Medicine has advanced so far, yet there are many limits to what we know and can do.

I recounted this story to my friend. She sat across from me reticently and, after a long pause, said, "What you do is incredibly hard."

I began to minimize what I did, and she stopped me. She

said I should take some time to reflect on what I do and its impact on me.

As I started my sabbatical, I sensed I was wounded. I felt broken and unsure if I would be ready to return to the emergency department. As a veteran, I was familiar with PTSD and PTSS. Thinking back to my psychiatric rotation in medical school, most of what I recalled was flashbacks and insomnia. Aside from the night shift disruptions, I slept well and never had what I considered a flashback. Yet, I sensed there was probably more to learn about PTSS and PTSD and began reading books on the topic. While very comfortable with the "trauma" of the gunshot, knife, and blunt variety- emotional trauma was not something I understood or identified with experiencing. Yet, there was a profound pull to learn everything I could.

I read *What Happened to You* by Oprah Winfrey and Dr. Bruce Perry. While I learned many things from this book, one of the most important concepts is that trauma is a universal human experience. No one, no matter how privileged, gets through life without suffering, at minimum, little "ts" or traumas. I consider most of my life traumas to be little to medium Ts.

Given the lack of what I consider a big T, I've been disappointed these traumas still profoundly affect me. Oprah's book helped me understand these traumas, especially when experienced when we're young, can leave large wounds. It is hard to know how to process them. The most powerful message is that we can recover. Following the pandemic, I didn't know if I could recover. I felt so depleted and wounded I didn't think there was a way to come back to emergency medicine. Yet, at the end of the book, they introduce the concept of posttraumatic growth.

Posttraumatic growth is a theory defined by the American Psychological Association as a transformation following trauma. This is not some quaint "everything happens for a reason" crap. To be clear, any trauma affects us, and we'd prefer it didn't happen. Yet, shit (trauma) happens. Until we get those magic wands, we can't make the past go poof. Accepting the experiences is not about absolving people who perpetrated acts of violence or aggression. As a friend once said, you may discover explanations for what happened or why someone did something, and they are simply explanations. The reason is not an excuse for what happened.

A cautionary note on looking for explanations: Consider how much time and what your expectations are related to finding an answer. Looking for explanations is rooted in closure. When I know why x happened, then I'll have closure and can begin to heal. It's perilous to link your healing to an external event. When searching for closure, the seeking may result in disappointment and more questions—looking for the why behind what happened can become an obsession and get in the way of healing. Explanations can be helpful. This is a great situation to involve a therapist in, as they can help guide you on whether this is helping you heal or is a distraction from your real goals and desires.

Posttraumatic growth must be a choice. It is not about becoming consumed by past traumas, and avenging the wrongs of what happened isn't required to move on or live with trauma. Moving on is also a euphemism. Some days, I feel like I've moved on from the pandemic. On other days, a doctor friend recounts going from room to room, holding up an iPad as she was in full PPE, for the final moments of far too many patients, and I'm crying and walking with her through those trauma fields. As my coach, Sharee Johnson, says, these traumas won't disappear. They will be part of the patchwork of our lives; over time, they will find their way into the quilt more proportionately. For the first years after the pandemic, it held a more outsized place in the quilt; it will always be prominent, ragged, and visible. But I am confident that the edges will soften.

Maybe you're still wondering what trauma is. I like Faith Harper's definition in *How to Unf*ck Your Brain*. She defines trauma in refreshingly simple terms: It's something that kicked your ass. This definition invites you to decide what has affected you without comparison or judgment. Physicians often compare their traumas, thinking that their experiences are somehow less significant than others. It's a dangerous practice that we need to let go of. Trauma isn't a competition; it's a deeply personal experience that affects everyone differently. There is no Olympics of trauma; we don't need to compare or rank our experiences.

Bessel van der Kolk's *The Body Keeps the Score* emphasizes that our bodies don't distinguish between small or big traumas. The body reacts based on its unique responses. Processing, or lack thereof, also depends on our support system. What may be a little t, when lacking the support of a loving family or, in medicine, a team, can morph into a more significant T.

We can't wholly untangle our personal and professional lives. Things that happen to us personally can lead to potential triggers for us professionally. It doesn't mean we can't be doctors, but we should explore these and process them to show up to work as our best selves.

One such experience for me involves a car accident. During the final week of medical school, a drunk driver T-boned my vehicle, resulting in it being totaled. Fortunately, I exited the car unharmed. I chose not to go to the hospital, partly influenced by my upcoming career in emergency medicine and the belief that I could self-assess my condition.

Then, I didn't fully comprehend the impact of that incident on me. Over time, I developed significant hypervigilance, particularly when other vehicles approached me from the left side. This anxiety intensified during my years of working at a trauma center, where I cared for severely injured patients, often from motor vehicle accidents. It became clear how a seemingly minor car accident, one I walked away from physically unharmed, could trigger post-traumatic stress symptoms, particularly when exacerbated by the demands of caring for such patients in my profession. This experience underscores how our personal lives can intersect with our professional roles. You don't have to navigate these challenges alone.

For me, like many people, my therapy started with psychotherapy, aka "talk therapy." A frequent criticism of therapy is that "it's just talk" and that people can spend years going to therapy and talking about the same things with little, if any, improvement. Especially for trauma, it is increasingly recognized that talk therapy may worsen PTSS and PTSD due to the reliving of the trauma. There are several emerging forms of therapy, and my therapist recommended Eye Movement Desensitization Reprocessing (EMDR). The central concept of EMDR is that traumas live in our bodies, not just inside our minds. Rapid eye movements are used to reprocess these traumas and to heal.

EMDR was discovered by Dr. Francine Shapiro and is based on the Adaptive Information Processing (AIP) model. The premise is that traumatic experiences disrupt the usual memory process and can create disconnections with language, sight, and hearing. To use an analogy from Dr. Katrina Landa, our brain has a "wound," and this damaged area is more susceptible to "injury" from new traumas. EMDR is not like wiping a hard drive. We still have memories; instead, the reprocessing helps the individual relate to the trauma differently.

For example, I still remember the car accident with my dad. I also remember the patients with traumatic injuries I've taken care of throughout my career. My reaction and how my body feels when I think about these things is different and less reactive.

I encourage all readers to be proactive when seeking mental health support. Just as healthcare is grappling with staffing shortages, so is the mental health community. It takes time to find the right therapist, and when you're in a challenging emotional or mental health event, it's hard to have the energy and clarity to find the best therapist. Given the amount of trauma we experience at work, we should have access to free and quality mental health support.

I look forward to a day when psychologists and other mental health professionals are embedded in our healthcare teams to attend to healthcare workers. I envision them helping with debriefs and other group facilitation, as well as one-on-one sessions that help with trauma processing and skill development to sustain us in this challenging profession.

Along with our jobs, many of us endured emotional trauma in childhood. *Buy Yourself the F*cking Lilies: And Other Rituals to Fix Your Life, from Someone Who's Been There* by Tara Schuster, helped me confront the family trauma I had experienced. It made me realize that specific childhood traumas I had downplayed could be reactivated when working with patients. I learned these early traumas needed to be processed, and although it has been a challenging journey, I'm grateful for my progress.

The Wounded Healer by Dr. Omar Reda explains how trauma impacts caregivers. Dr. Reda's thesis is that caregiving involves being wounded. Many of us build emotional walls or what Dr. Brené Brown calls armor. We armor up before entering our workplaces, thinking we can keep those traumas at bay. However, what became apparent in 2021 was that before my deployment in 2016, I used to cry freely and found it cathartic. I would even intentionally watch emotional movies to have a good cry. Yet, during deployment, I stopped crying altogether, even when faced with things that would have easily made me cry before. This emotional suppression continued when I moved to Los Angeles and became more apparent as I felt hardened by the volume and severity of the trauma I encountered.

Dr. Reda's book served as a reminder that our work affects us, and that's not something negative. We are more whole when we acknowledge our vulnerability and the emotional toll caregiving can take. I want to emphasize the impact of going into our work fully armored, with the mindset that nothing will affect us. We might believe we can disconnect from our professional experiences by numbing out once we get home. However, what we may not realize is that over the years, this emotional detachment builds up trauma residues within us. Dr. Dan Dworkis from Mission Critical Teams introduced me to the idea that our experiences leave residues on us. By 2021, I had accumulated ten years' worth of this residue, and it became clear that I needed to pause and process them during my three-month sabbatical.

I also listened to Dr. Brené Brown's episode on *Unlocking Us*, where she talks about her sabbatical, which deeply resonated with me. She used the phrase "going out horizontally instead of vertically," which encapsulated how I felt about 2021. I, too, felt like I had gone out horizontally, as there was no other choice but to halt and focus on getting healthy before returning.

When you need breaks, whether short respites or extended sabbaticals, try to take them while standing up. Don't wait until you're emotionally and physically drained to where you have no other option but to stop abruptly.

However, if you find yourself at that breaking point, that is also an excellent time to take the break and save yourself the self-flagellation of not taking the break earlier.

In this book's final round of editing, I read Stephanie Foo's book, *What My Bones Know*. In her harrowing and raw narrative of surviving childhood abuse, she shares her diagnosis of Complex PTSD and her path to recovery. I am convinced that many healthcare professionals also have complex PTSD or PTSS. As the name implies, it is complex and emerges after prolonged and many traumatic events, which happen disproportionately to healthcare professionals and veterans. Unlike classic PTSD, the triggers become more numerous and more difficult to unravel.

One of the key symptoms of complex PTSD is an emotional flashback. While the experience of an emotional flashback can vary, some describe it as an overwhelming emotion that is inescapable and may pop up without an apparent reason (common when triggers are multiple and tied to many events). It's beyond the scope of this book for me to explain Complex PTSD. Yet, I find it very important to share that it exists so we understand it for patients and our colleagues. It is still (as of the writing of this book) not recognized in the DSM-5, the bible of psychiatric diagnoses. This leads to so many people not being correctly diagnosed.

Returning to how long it takes to recover- it is a process.

It is an active choice to keep recovering. Learning about complex PTSD and PTSS expanded my understanding of what trauma is and the profound impact it has on our brains. It also gave me new techniques and the hope that recovery could occur. Stephanie Foo's book also helped me understand why I stopped crying. I was numbing and detaching. I couldn't even realize that I was doing it. It felt like crying had just left my emotional range for a few years. At first, I told myself that it was a good sign. I wasn't so "soft" anymore.

Many times, people have asked me how I knew I was improving. For a long time, I had a hard time answering the question. Now, I know that one of the leading indicators was the ability to cry again. I'm back to watching a movie and needing the tissues close by! I don't always cry, but I allow myself to be moved again. I feel like in my younger years, primarily due to not having great role modeling on how to move through difficult emotions, when they came, they were like a wave that I wasn't sure I would come out the other side of. It took the sabbatical, a complete surrender to the wave, to come out the other side.

When I talk to doctors, they often won't consider a sabbatical or pause due to financial reasons. Student loans, among other things we acquire, make us feel like we can't stop working. Your career is a marathon. Walking or taking a breather is allowed. You can't finish the race if you're not alive. The unprocessed trauma that many of us carry is killing us emotionally and physically.

In addition to the financial reasons, physicians are penalized for taking breaks. Resume gaps are viewed with high levels of scrutiny and require written explanations, which will often delay obtaining clinical credentials. Rather than shaming physicians, yet again, for taking breaks, the medical culture desperately needs to embrace and applaud these breaks as part of being a human and, yes, a doctor. Even a break of less than one week between my graduation from medical school and moving to California required an explanation. This is simply absurd and undoubtedly contributes to the feeling that we can't take breaks.

You deserve rest and recovery. Support is available from friends, colleagues, mental health professionals, and coaches. There are many individuals out there who can help you in your journey. Remember, it's your life. Only you have the complete picture of what you need and what will fill your cup, and nobody else will do it for you.

Reflect:

After reading about the journey through burnout, moral injury, and personal trauma, what experiences resonate with you, and how have you addressed or navigated them?

_____

_____

_____

Reimagine:

Considering the concept of post-traumatic growth, how can you envision transforming your most challenging experiences into opportunities for personal development and more profound understanding?

_____

_____

_____

_____

Respond:

What steps can you take to reconnect with your passion and commitment towards your personal and professional life, drawing inspiration from the resilience and recovery journey shared in the chapter?

_____

_____

_____

_____

Resources:

What Happened to You?: Conversations on Trauma, Resilience, and Healing by Bruce Perry and Oprah Winfrey.

The Body Keeps the Score: Brain, Mind, and Body in the Healing of Trauma by Sean Pratt, Bessel A. van der Kolk, et al.

How to Unf*ck Your Brain by Faith Harper.

The Wounded Healer: The Pain of and Joy of Caregiving by Omar Reda

Buy Yourself the F*cking Lilies: And Other Rituals to Fix Your Life, from Someone Who's Been There by Tara Schuster

What My Bones Know by Stephanie Foo

Getting Past Your Past: Take Control of Your Life with Self-Help Techniques from EMDR Therapy by Francine Shapiro.

For more about how your physical heart works and how it is interconnected with emotional well-being, read:

Just One Heart: A Cardiologist's Guide to Healing, Health and Happiness by Jonathan Fisher.

Michelle Woolhouse's *The Wonder Within: A heart-led playbook for the anxious, stressed, and burnt out.* You can also listen to Bridging the Gap: Integrating Ancient Wisdom with Modern Science in Healthcare- Dr. Michelle Woolhouse, episode 45 of the *Heartline* podcast.

CHAPTER 11

THE DOCTOR GOES TO THE DOCTOR

"It's so important, too…for physicians to take care of themselves because how can you teach someone how to do something that you're not doing?" — Dr. Danielle Douglas, on Heartline podcast, Oct 24, 2023

As an emergency medicine physician, seeking medical care for myself can be challenging. After spending years working in the bustling emergency department environment, my initial instinct leans towards downplaying any symptoms I might experience, telling myself, "These symptoms are probably minor." I usually question whether I must consult another physician.

Like many others, I also gained weight during the pandemic. Despite trying to shed those extra pounds using various methods, I faced several obstacles. During one of my conversations with a colleague from the emergency department, I learned about the prevalence of this issue, particularly among individuals in high-stress professions. Excess cortisol production can significantly contribute to weight gain in such demanding roles.

This colleague generously shared her extensive

knowledge concerning cortisol, hormonal balance, nutrition, and the intricate connection between the mind and body, which piqued my interest. She had completed a functional medicine fellowship and opened a private practice. After some initial procrastination, I eventually mustered the courage to contact her.

Her approach was firmly grounded in the principles of personalized and optimized health. She emphasized the pivotal role of gut health and detoxification pathways, gradually shifting toward lifestyle changes encompassing dietary improvements, meditation, and regular exercise. As a physician, I particularly resonated with functional medicine's commitment to scientific evidence and its incorporation of comprehensive lab work.

The work-up included a 24-hour salivary cortisol test. Cortisol levels show a daily rhythm, requiring multiple salivary samples to construct a correct cortisol curve throughout the day. This data-driven approach aligned perfectly with my penchant for evidence.

After receiving the results, I was presented with a visual representation of my cortisol curve, which appeared at first glance normal, save for one glaring problem: my cortisol levels were alarmingly low. I was producing a mere 1% of the cortisol typically expected for an individual of my age and sex. This revelation struck me with an intense emotional jolt. It was a visual representation of the chronic stress I had endured. I teared up as it mirrored how I felt: tired and like I had no energy to keep going.

The prolonged and relentless stress stemming from my medical residency, deployment experiences, the intensity of clinical work post-deployment, and the additional burden of the pandemic had taken a heavy toll on my adrenal glands. They had reached a point where they could no longer sustain the demand for cortisol production.

My functional medicine physician advised me to prioritize recovery over rigorous physical activities such as running a half marathon. Instead, she recommended meditation, yoga, and gentle strength training as more suitable options until I regained my strength and overall health.

Earlier, I mentioned the many gaps in our medical understanding. Western medicine, which emphasizes medications and downplays lifestyle interventions that optimize sleep, social connection, and diet, also contributes to these gaps. Functional medicine flips the equation and emphasizes that food is medicine. We create a lot of false dichotomies. It's not either Western medicine or functional medicine. It's both.

It is common for emergency department patients to present after they have exhausted Western medicine's capability. Maybe they have chronic abdominal pain, and they've had CTs, MRIs, endoscopies, pill cameras, and more in search of an answer. Functional medicine is a great avenue to consider when you're curious about more ways of evaluating and treating health conditions.

Recognizing that variations in my sleep were unavoidable when working in emergency medicine, I began to use the Oura ring to provide objective feedback on my sleep. The device helps me see when I'm in the "red" and have not recovered and lets me adjust my schedule to add more rest. Over time, I can predict when I will need more time to recover and proactively schedule it. For example, if I'm still fatigued the second day after a night shift, sleeping later and engaging in lighter cognitive activities that day help with recovery.

When I consulted with Dr. Danielle regarding my health, she began with questions to assess to what degree I had addressed my trauma history. She underscored the significance of tackling the root cause, which for many people is unresolved emotional trauma. She was adamant about the importance of starting trauma interventions as the key to unlocking physical well-being. Fortunately, I had embarked on this journey of trauma processing for about a year.

When we reflect on what we do in medicine, it is

incredible. From surgeons who can operate for hours on end, in some cases, literally holding their breath to avoid any excess movement when placing a microsuture to a physician juggling the chaos of a busy emergency department, these are Olympic-level challenges to the mind and body. Physicians and surgeons deserve individualized plans to optimize sleep, nutrition, and physical activity. The long hours, sleep disturbances, and ergonomic challenges we face are all examples of occupational stressors that can have significant morbidity and even mortality implications. Many physicians work as independent contractors, with no scheduled breaks, family leave, paid sick time, or other protections that our nursing and other allied health professionals have through an employed model subject to labor laws.

While functional medicine has proved to be an excellent formula for my health journey, many practitioners and philosophies can support your well-being. On a past episode of the *Heartline* podcast, I interviewed Dr. Raquel Harrison, founder of Acute 2 Root (www.acute2root.com). In this episode, she shared her journey to becoming board-certified in Lifestyle Medicine. She discussed the six pillars of lifestyle medicine: A whole-food, plant-predominant eating pattern, physical activity, restorative sleep, stress management, avoidance of risky behaviors, and positive social connections.

Over the past few years, I've gained an appreciation for the seasonal component of well-being. This manifests in several ways in my life. First, we eat more seasonally. I grew up eating food primarily bought at the grocery store. In many grocery stores, the food preset is shipped in from around the world. Now, we have a large garden and a small orchard. With the changing of the seasons, the food in our backyard changes. I look forward to the first peas of the season each spring. These vibrant green peas have a firm texture and taste nothing like the mushy, green-brown blah I grew up eating from a can. The summertime brings tomatoes, and there's this period from July-August that is stone fruit season (peaches, nectarines, other fruits with a pit, aka stone); then we move into figs, and the start of fall brings us pomegranates and squash. Winter is citrus season. Eating seasonally adds variation to what we eat, which keeps us out of a food rut. Food shipped long distances is under-ripe, doesn't taste as good, and is nutritionally less dense.

In addition to this seasonal eating, I incorporate seasonality into my fitness routine. In the summer, I paddleboard and swim more. In the winter (since I live in San Diego), I hike more, as our days are cooler, and the summertime can be too hot to hike safely. Varying the workouts also prevents monotony and gets me outside more when I work with and not against the natural variation in the seasons.

Social connections are a powerful predictor of well-being. Cultivate connections beyond a romantic partner. Quality relationships with colleagues, friends, and family are essential for developing a social support network. Research shows that our fulfillment from work increases with workplace friendships.[23] Some workplace friendships will transverse the workplace, which is beautiful but unnecessary for improved well-being. There are many colleagues I don't socialize with outside of work, but their smiles and short, friendly exchanges on shift are welcome reprieves from a challenging day. These interactions can trigger the release of oxytocin, the hormone (aka the love hormone) that we feel when we're close to someone, such as during a hug. Moments like a warm exchange that triggers oxytocin are examples of leveraging the tend-and-befriend response. This is an underreported stress response compared to fight or flight, which gets the most attention. Appropriately cultivating the tend-and-befriend response is crucial to navigating challenging moments in life.

In addition to work colleagues, I have a strong network of self-care professionals who provide meaningful connections. My chiropractor always greets me, "Hey doc, how's it going?" He acknowledges that I'm a doctor and asks how things are going, whether I'm working too much, and what trip I have coming up. These are brief exchanges but enhance connection.

My hair stylist for nearly ten years, Carmel Moreno, has provided unbelievable support and contributed to my growth. When I got the call that I was deploying, I was told I may leave the country in two weeks. As vain as it may be, I called Carmel and left a voicemail saying I wanted her to do my hair again before I left. My voice cracked as I was experiencing profound grief around all the people I wouldn't see for many months. When I showed up to get my hair done, she and her assistant had flowers and a meal waiting for me. Writing these words fills me with tears, and the impact of that act of kindness and the connection it created in us was profound.

Later, Carmel would tell me about EMDR, and while I wouldn't seek it out, years later, when I finally found it, our bond again strengthened as I would share with her the profound healing it provided. While I know not everyone will be as fortunate or need the support of a hair stylist, as a woman, I feel that our hair is more than just hair. When I came home from deployment, I was so drained. Sitting in Carmel's chair, I said, "Cut it out. Cut out the deployment." While I didn't shave my head, she cut a substantial amount of hair because I felt it was holding so much pain. The energy was dull, and I needed my head lightened from its load.

When I returned from deployment, I was the skinniest I had ever been. Later, when Carmel and I would talk about that period, she said, "You didn't look healthy. You looked fragile." Having people in our lives who can see, over time, through the ups and downs lets them have real insight into how we're doing. So many people said, "You look great." Carmel could see behind the outward facade of thinness.

While I pay my chiropractor, my hair stylist, and yes, my functional medicine doctor, paying for something doesn't always have to stop at that transaction. The connections outlined transform everyday interactions into meaningful connections. Even my dry cleaner is a source of connection. The mundane act of dropping my dry cleaning is altered by, "Hi, Dr. Andrea, it's great to see you." Beyond removing the stains on my lab coat, I'm buoyed by her kindness and admiration.

For now, the best many of us can do is to individually seek a support team to guide us in our journeys to be healthier in an unhealthy system. We must do this work individually to restore the energy to make the main changes needed to the system. We can't pour from an empty cup.

Reflect:

What is an area of your health and well-being in which you desire true optimization rather than simply the absence of illness or injury?

_____

_____

_____

_____

Reimagine:

What would your life look like if you reached this optimized state of well-being or health?

_____

_____

_____

_____

Respond:

What is one action you're willing to take to start this journey?

_____

_____

_____

_____

Resources:

The Institute for Functional Medicine: www.ifm.org

American College of Lifestyle Medicine. https://lifestylemedicine.org/

Oura ring (www.ouraring.com) and other wearable devices can provide helpful physiological information to improve your well-being.

Arena Labs (www.arenalabs.co) is a leader in next-level individual and organizational practices that support improved performance. They also provide support on wearable technology and how to leverage the data provided to improve well-being.

Andrea Austin

CHAPTER 12

VALUES, BOUNDARIES, AND PRIORITIES

"Boundaries are not rules for other people, but rules for ourselves. It's what I'm going to do if this happens. — Dr. Shideh Shafie, on the Heartline podcast, Mar 5, 2024

Imagine you're at work, and everything that could go wrong is going wrong. You are three patients behind, the electronic medical record is on downtime, and there are two callouts, further stressing the department. At that moment, the massage you had earlier in the day or the self-care planned for tomorrow does not provide the help you desperately need. So, what's the alternative? What can you turn to in such demanding situations?

While our work is inherently stressful, it's also full of meaning and purpose. How do we embrace the stress and have the tools to navigate it in the moment? After trying everything else, the long-term fix has been aligning my values, priorities, and boundaries.

What are your values? Let's start with an exercise. Review the table below and select the top 10 values that speak to you. The key is to pick the words that are meaningful and ring true to you, not the words that you think you ***should choose*** based on the expectations of others.

Integrity	Authenticity	Innovation
Honesty	Loyalty	Creativity
Respect	Optimism	Curiosity
Responsibility	Wisdom	Growth
Compassion	Self-discipline	Self-awareness
Empathy	Justice	
Gratitude	Fairness	Self-improvement
Kindness	Tolerance	Balance
Aesthetics	Acceptance	Harmony
Generosity	Open-mindedness	Environmental stewardship
Courage		
Perseverance	Equality	Graciousness
Humility	Teamwork	Spirituality
Patience	Cooperation	Service
Forgiveness	Flexibility	

Once you get ten circled, then put checkmarks next to your top five. There's debate among experts around how many guiding values one can or should have. I'd recommend two to three core values. If you struggle to pick your top two to three, you likely need more time to sit with what resonates most strongly with you. Journaling, talking with friends and loved ones, or a coach can help you reflect on what is most true. These will provide the overarching values you can turn to for the big decisions and challenging moments in life. You may notice a conflict between the values when you get beyond two or three. While this is common, as we're complex, multifaceted beings, it helps to have the two to three that are most salient for you.

Awareness of the other values that resonate with you is helpful because when you feel a strong emotion, there may be a value farther down your list that underpins the feeling. On further reflection, you may recognize a value further down your list being challenged. For example, aesthetics comes in at number eight on my list of values. I like our yard to have a particular look and feel, and I have become irritable during some home improvement projects. The last time it happened, I realized that aesthetics matter to me. I like art, style, creating a vibe, and periods of construction challenges that temporarily. I know this now, and I can better communicate this to my husband.

After you get it down to two or three, return to these words over the next few months. Write them down on sticky notes and have ready access to review them at work, at home, and in many situations. Do they ring true across all aspects of your life? We believe in core values, and we can live according to them despite our situations.

Another interesting exercise to explore your values is to fill out your Ikigai. Ikigai is a Japanese word for a reason to live. In the exercise below, fill in what you love, what the world needs, what you are good at, and what you can be paid for. Working towards that magic overlap of all four is the Ikigai! When considering what activities fall in the Ikigai, what values underpin them? As an intelligent, capable person, I know many things may fall under an Ikigai. Ponder why you are pursuing them and consider how they relate to your core values.

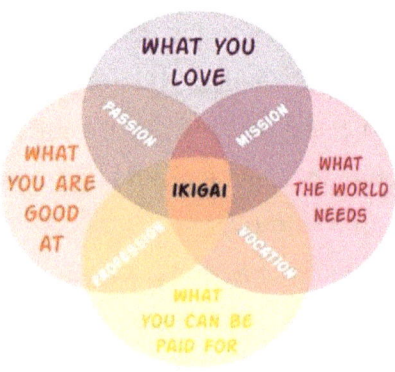

Image credit: Iva - stock.adobe.com

I frequently felt that my values, boundaries, and priorities were mismatched in medicine and the military. Both medicine and the military are marked by strict hierarchies and specific requirements to progress, whether that means advancing to the following year in residency or achieving a higher rank. As I started this new phase, one where I had real choices about where I worked and what I pursued, I began to experience a sense of unease. It raised questions like: What do I truly desire? Why do I want it? What holds genuine importance?

Values serve as guiding principles in our lives, representing what we hold dear and essential. They offer invaluable assistance when faced with decisions. After many months of reflection and refinement, I landed on:

1. **Innovation**: Given my specialization in simulation within education, I thrive when I can create new advancements. Medicine generally moves slowly, and many cultures within medicine are slow to adopt change and very hierarchical, making it harder to "break in" and innovate. In simulation, I can move quickly to iterate on an issue or problem without risk to patients while aligning with my core value of innovation.

2. **Meaningful Work**: I'm drawn to institutions with a greater purpose beyond merely delivering healthcare and generating profits. I've felt the most energy

around service-driven organizations and entities. For example, military healthcare focuses on providing excellent healthcare to the nation's service members.

At LA County, the patient population was loved. A patient population that included many homeless patients. I'll never forget watching a team of nurses and residents care for an injured patient experiencing homelessness. He was covered in dirt and bugs, and the smell was inescapable. At the top of the bed, one of the residents stood leading the resuscitation, and she had towels wrapped around his head to provide a cushion. She spoke softly and caringly to him, explaining what everyone was doing. I distinctly remember feeling a profound awe and admiration for the team and the excellent work.

3. **Autonomy**: I relish having control over my body, mind, and schedule, along with the independence to practice medicine and teach in a way that aligns with my values. However, I find working in places that are overly reliant on protocols, inflexible, and resistant to advancements in medicine and education dissatisfying.

It took about one year after I departed from the military for my values to become apparent. It became clear that my initial job choices conflicted with these values. Many challenges and a sense of uncertainty marked this period. By directing my focused attention toward my values, I restructured my work to revolve around them, focusing on what nourishes me emotionally and intellectually.

A boundary, as defined by the dictionary, is a line that demarcates the limits of a particular area—a dividing line. Boundaries are a fundamental human requirement and a fundamental right. We all require certain boundaries, such as the right to be free from unwanted physical contact. Still, medical education systematically erodes boundaries. For example, we have little control over our schedules during clinical rotations. On my surgery rotation, it was common to arrive at the hospital by 5 a.m. and leave around 6 or 7 p.m. each night, with barely enough time to address basic human needs like eating and sleeping. These fundamental requirements are suppressed and disregarded.

As Dr. Shideh Shafie reminds us, the key is not just establishing the boundary; it's developing a plan for what you will do when violated. The rest of the world, while it would be so wonderful if they didn't test our boundaries...the truth is they will get tested a lot! Especially as a doctor! For example, what will I do when the scheduler reaches out and asks me to work more shifts than I am comfortable working? Have a plan that may be as simple as creating space and time to respond. One of my favorite replies is, "Thank you, I'll get back to you."

Boundaries are akin to strengthening your muscles to lift heavier weights. At first, it can be difficult, and you might feel shaky. However, don't let momentary wavering deter you from standing your ground. With practice, holding boundaries becomes more accessible. Additionally, I've discovered that following through on your boundaries discourages future undesirable behavior.

Dr. Shafie also explained the concept of internal boundaries, which are promises we make to ourselves. These have been decimated during the medical education process. One of my internal boundaries is that I like to start my mornings leisurely two to three days per week, especially on Sundays. This involves making coffee, curling up on the couch, and cuddling with my dogs for 30-45 minutes. Going to the gym, choir lessons, or your child's sports or music performances are examples of promises we make to ourselves. While we need to be flexible, we must treat ourselves with as much courtesy as a friend. How would you respond to a friend that keeps cancelling on you? This slight mindset shift that you will honor yourself and your commitments and internal boundaries as much as you would making an appointment to see a friend can shift your entire life.

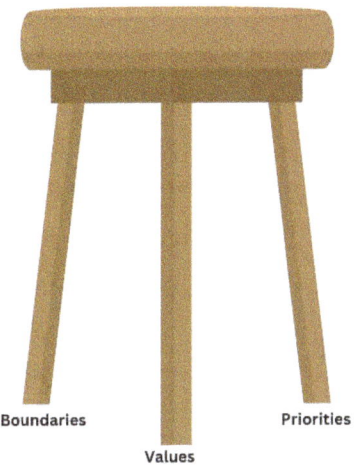

Boundaries   Priorities

Values

Image credit: Adapted from original by Jeronimo Ramos - stock.adobe.com

The third important part, akin to the third leg of a stool, is priorities. Medical professionals continually grapple with competing priorities that demand our attention. Throughout your career, your priorities are guaranteed to undergo significant shifts. Early on, you might be heavily focused on your work, while later, the need to set aside more time for family and personal life becomes paramount. We miss many family and friend events during medical school and residency, and many of us desire to "catch up." Your values remain steadfast, serving as unwavering guideposts through life's ups and downs. Priorities, however, let you adapt and address emerging goals and necessities in your professional and personal spheres.

Exercise: Draw your stool with the length of each leg,

representing your clarity on the following categories: values, boundaries, and priorities. Is your stool really short? Is your stool lopsided (values with a long leg, but boundaries and values short)? Hence, you've got a super lopsided stool that won't handle any weight or stress. This is how a lot of us walk around. Life hits us so hard because we don't have the clarity of a solid stool to shoulder the stress.

If you find yourself on the brink of burnout and realize that self-care and vacations alone aren't enough for your recovery, consider dedicating time to articulate your values, boundaries, and priorities. Then, start documenting how you currently allocate your time. With a spirit of curiosity and letting go of judgment, do you observe any areas of misalignment? What's one step to bring your life into better harmony? Sometimes, it's not about upending your existence (although occasionally necessary); it could be as straightforward as reframing your perspective. Perhaps many aspects of your day align with your values, boundaries, and priorities, but you still need to acknowledge this alignment consciously. Recognizing how these challenges fit into your broader plan, harmonizing with a priority, might help you tolerate them more effectively. For example, meeting the demanding criteria for the associate professor position could align with your value of service and desire to serve as a role model for aspiring women in academia. However, pursuing the associate professorship might not make sense if you closely examine your values and priorities. There may be an opportunity to hit the pause button and reassess your priorities.

I have a desire for justice and service. I can get swept up in the excitement, outrage, or other emotions to overextend myself and get involved in various causes. In these cases, returning to my Ikigai is essential. What does the world need, what am I good at, and is there fair compensation for the work? There are many things I get moved by, or I feel "should" get done. My friend and colleague, Dr. Gerald Platt, once shared with me how he was on his way home from work and saw a fire on the side of the road. He thought, "Oh wow, I should do something." Then, he saw the fire trucks and thought, "It's not my fire." He applied that phrase to several issues that would come up that were not his responsibility or that he didn't have the resources to tackle: It's not my fire. As someone who gets quickly fired up, telling myself regularly, "It's not my fire," has kept me from getting burned many times.

The other breakthrough concept that has helped me focus on my involvement in potential opportunities is a framework Susannah Fox provides in her book *Rebel Health: A Field Guide to the Patient-Led Revolution in Medical Care*. She describes four archetypes of changemakers in healthcare: the seeker, networker, solver, and champion. Somewhere along the way, I became a networker. It stems from my love of people and stories. I don't see networking as the climbing or the ambitious angle associated with it. Instead, networking is about connecting people. I also love the efficiency of networking. Life and healthcare are complex! I get immense joy from connecting people and watching the solution or fix emerge from the connection between two people.

Sharee Johnson, a psychologist and coach who works with physicians, consistently reminds me that our boundaries and priorities are not fixed. Our lives are in perpetual flux, and while our values, once deeply explored, usually remain relatively constant, our boundaries and priorities can undergo significant shifts. I tolerated various things in my 20s that no longer align with my preferences in my 30s. For example, sharing a room was not a big deal in my 20s. However, as I approach my 40s, having a roommate at this phase of life is not something I would choose. As an ambivert, a blend of introvert and extrovert traits, I relish my extroverted interactions with people during the day. But then, I require about 1-2 hours of solitude before bedtime to gather my thoughts and recharge. I am confident there will be a day when working weekends and nights will not be a boundary that I will allow to be traversed. Our boundaries are allowed to change. This is a radical idea for medical administrators and fellow doctors.

The transformation of us as both individuals and collectively to transform healthcare begins with boundaries.

The erosion of boundaries regarding compensation, sleep, and resources, including appropriate staffing, efficient electronic medical records, and so on, is at the heart of the dysfunction in medicine. A surgeon will only start a case with the appropriate staff, lighting, and tools to perform surgery. We constantly bootstrap in the emergency department and many other healthcare settings. Bootstrapping refers to dealing with a situation with the current resources. While bootstrapping is rooted in a healthy work ethic and ingenuity, bootstraps snap, harming us as individual clinicians and, long-term, our patients.

Bootstrapping can lead to moral injury. When I began my emergency medicine residency, seeing a patient in the waiting room was nearly unheard of. Mostly, patients were seen in rooms with exam tables or beds. This was important, as many chief complaints warrant patients being in a gown to evaluate rashes or signs of trauma and to lie down to perform a proper abdominal exam. Over the last few years, as the primary care system continues to collapse and more patients pour into the emergency department, we have begun to let the boundary of seeing patients in beds fall to the wayside. Now, I will submit that only some people need a bed. Some "vertical" medicine, i.e., keeping patients in a chair versus a bed, is reasonable. Yet, many patients don't get a proper abdominal exam. Because we don't have a place to perform serial exams, we order a CT scan of the abdomen. This is the reality of waiting room medicine. The moral injury comes with knowing that we're not performing the careful and serial exams we were trained to do, and we are also ordering more CTs than are needed. Waiting room medicine usually involves rushed care and interviews in suboptimal locations for comfort and privacy. This also contributes to our moral injury.

Waiting room medicine is something I tolerate, as every emergency department I work in does it. If I set the boundary of no waiting room medicine, I would need to leave our specialty. That day may come, just not yet. I'm still in the fight, and sharing the story of moral injury in the emergency department, like waiting room medicine, can transform our specialty. I haven't given up on emergency medicine, but I also honor my internal boundaries. I can't work full-time in this specialty. It hurts my heart too much. I can do about two days in a row, and then I need a few days off to rest, write, and do the changemaking work I believe will decrease the bootstrapping and moral injury we endure. I also know a day may come when my heart hurts too much, and that's okay, too. We may evolve, and I know there will be more changemakers behind me.

Reflect:

What are examples of things that no longer align with your values, boundaries, or priorities?

_____

_____

_____

Reimagine:

How would your life differ if you honor your values, boundaries, or priorities?

_____

_____

_____

Respond:

What's a manageable step to solidify this promise to yourself, to honor the specific value, boundary, or priority you've outlined?

_____

_____

_____

Resources:

The Power of No: Learning to Establish Boundaries as a Physician with Dr. Shideh Shafie. Episode 66 of the *Heartline* podcast.

Boundaries: 124. How to Say No: Boundaries with Nedra Glover Tawwab *We Can Do Hard Things* podcast.

CHAPTER 13

AGENCY AS THE ANTIDOTE TO A FAILING HEALTHCARE SYSTEM

"We do have agency, and I would challenge that physicians have a lot more agency than we are owning right now…we should be harnessing that for good and working to change the system." —
Dr. Andrea Austin, on Heartline podcast, Nov 15, 2022

In Dr. Christina Maslach's classic definition of burnout, three elements come into play: exhaustion, depersonalization, and decreased personal efficacy. Personal efficacy refers to one's ability to produce the desired or intended result, and it is influenced by both objective and subjective factors affecting one's capacity to achieve a particular outcome.

Reflecting on the healthcare landscape during the pandemic, it felt like we were amidst a relentless tide of COVID-19 patients, with the healthcare system struggling to meet the needs of patients and healthcare workers. I experienced a profound sense of reducing efficacy. It was as if I had become trapped in a healthcare version of the Sisyphus myth, relentlessly pushing the boulder of patient care up the hill of our dysfunctional healthcare system.

According to psychological literature, the antithesis of

self-efficacy or agency is what psychology terms "learned helplessness." Learned helplessness was first identified in 1967 based on experiments with dogs exposed to inescapable shocks, which later led them to give up on escaping shocks when they had the opportunity to do so. Studies by Linzer and Visser have found that maintaining a sense of control over one's work, which is closely linked to autonomy, is pivotal in preventing burnout among physicians.[24]

A later paper in 1978 further delineates learned helplessness in people as two types: 1) Personal and 2) Universal in the framework of attributional learned helplessness.[25] Applying these terms to the context of emergency medicine work by physicians, an example of personal learned helplessness is, "There's nothing I can do to improve the flow in our emergency department. Every time I try, I get shot down. I don't have the skills to make any changes. Maybe if I got an MBA, it would be better." An example of universal learned helplessness is, "I can't improve flow in our emergency department. Without more staff, which costs more money, there aren't enough resources, and I can't change that. The system is broken."

Looking back, as much as it pains me to admit, I experienced learned helplessness, specifically of the universal variety. I had a reoccurring thought, "The system is screwed. It doesn't matter if I keep showing up."

Psychologists define learned helplessness as a phenomenon that occurs "when an individual continuously faces a negative, uncontrollable situation and stops trying to change their circumstances." Learned helplessness among physicians is rarely mentioned or described in the medical literature. George et al. described physicians as feeling like the "glue that binds together elements of a dysfunctional system..."[26] Being that glue had been part of my identity as an emergency doctor. If I wasn't the glue or felt a sense of pride being that glue, could I practice emergency medicine? Maybe leaving emergency medicine would remove me from the moral injury of having to explain to a woman with metastatic cancer and immunocompromised why she was waiting in a non-isolation room and likely getting exposed to many illnesses.

The concept of agency is related to self-efficacy, introduced by psychologist Dr. Albert Bandura. In an article by Bandura from 2001, he describes how social cognitive theory applies to agency. He identifies three types of agency, "direct personal agency, proxy agency that relies on others to act on one's behest to secure desired outcomes, and collective agency exercised through socially coordinative and interdependent effort."[27] This framework is beneficial when applied to physicians' roles in medicine, as that personal agency may feel high early in the career when applied to the ability to make changes for the individual patient. For example, feeling a high sense of agency when ordering a medication to relieve pain. Later in the career, when system-level problems become apparent and potentially the focus of some physicians' careers, the skills needed to impact collective agency are different and not always taught in medical school or residency.

Meanwhile, the excitement and sense of efficacy in doing the personal agency work of ordering medications and other doctoring tasks may seem less significant. Physicians will say, "I'm just a cog in this machine," or "I'm a burger flipper." This type of language is understandable (I've uttered similar words) yet surprising. We are highly skilled and doing meaningful work; we aren't easily replaceable. While there are many ways the system makes us feel like cogs- we aren't. We must recognize the thought distortion and acknowledge that it can reduce our sense of agency and self-efficacy.

While it seems small, our words matter. When we use language that minimizes our contributions, it has an effect. We react emotionally to "cog in the wheel" and the idea of being stuck, replaceable, or discounted. Remembering to create some distance in our thought by changing "I am a cog in this machine" to "I feel like a cog in this machine" is a powerful way to begin to recognize that we aren't cogs and that this is a feeling. Then, we can start to examine the evidence and reframe these thoughts.

> What if all the physicians didn't show up to work for a day?

This powerful thought experiment can help you rekindle your sense of agency. If it's hard for you to imagine no doctors showing up for work, consider the history of doctor strikes in Kenya.[28] A colleague was on the ground during one such strike and shared the chaos and horrors he saw. He shared that the Kenyan military had to be activated when patients, tragically, from a psychiatric hospital, were released to the streets. The stories of suffering are staggering, from babies left unattended in the NICU to the horror of trauma patients succumbing to their injuries; many would have been survivable with the swift actions of physicians. I am not suggesting that we go on strike. I use this example to help us channel the real sense of pride and profound agency we possess. Life is not a medical drama. People cannot step in and provide the level of care that physicians do swiftly every day.

***

Another tool to rekindle a sense of personal agency is to embrace the beginner's mindset. As an experienced physician, I find it easy to minimize the impact we have. Yet, from the beginner's viewpoint, the first time you successfully repair a laceration or diagnose a heart attack, there is a profound sense of efficacy. Being involved in medical education has helped me tremendously. Each day I teach medical students and residents, I am forced to see things from the beginner's viewpoint. Walking them through the procedures and diagnostic process that seem rote helps me know that I've come a long way and I still have a lot to give. If you don't work with medical students or residents, there are people around you to teach, including your patients. Nurses and other ancillary staff frequently want more explanations and appreciate a few moments explaining the diagnostic approach or therapeutic decisions. Often, EMS staff are eager for a few pearls or explanations for the initial treatment plan. Shifting the mindset from potential interruptions to opportunities to reconnect with yourself and your sense of agency and the ability to effect change within your clinical realm is essential.

The past few years have undeniably presented us with immense challenges, and healthcare professionals, including myself, have felt besieged by the hardships brought on by the pandemic and the broader issues within our healthcare systems. Despite enduring a relentless stream of challenges, I'm beginning to detect glimmers of resilience and determination that propel me to confront the formidable issues in healthcare.

The healthcare landscape is undeniably fraught with difficulties, and my experiences in the emergency department have laid bare the severity of these challenges.

Given the overwhelming influx of patients and the constraints of limited resources, there are moments when it seems nearly impossible to deliver adequate care. This dilemma has given rise to a profound sense of moral injury, exacting an emotional toll on healthcare professionals.

In Dr. Brené Brown's two-part Unlocking Us podcast interview featuring Anand Giridharadas, they dig into the pervasive despair and hopelessness permeating our society. Many individuals believe that the system is so profoundly fractured, immense in scale, and heavily influenced by powerful entities it appears unfixable, whether we're discussing our nation or the realm of healthcare.

In medicine, perceiving the system as an unchangeable behemoth is disheartening, especially when inequities and inefficiencies mar it. Some healthcare professionals even contemplate abandoning the field and exploring alternative career paths like real estate. While I wholeheartedly support those who make such choices for their well-being, I'm genuinely concerned about potentially losing expertise and dedication from seasoned healthcare workers.

Listening to Giridharadas, I was deeply struck by his assertion that despair is by design, and I find this sentiment particularly resonates within medicine. Some individuals reap significant benefits from the current system, capitalizing on the status quo. At the same time, healthcare professionals, particularly those on the front lines, grapple with alarmingly high rates of moral injury that fuel burnout, attrition, physician depression, anxiety, and even suicide.

Nevertheless, physicians, in particular, wield a substantial reservoir of expertise that can be harnessed to exert considerable agency for change. Our extensive training, coupled with the altruism that propelled many of us to pursue medicine, has the potential to be powerful drivers of transformation.

Yet starting change becomes a formidable challenge when we are overworked and burned out. Many things hinder us from harnessing our agency. Inherent to agency is action; you require time and energy to do anything. Thus, we must discuss what affects doctors' time and energy individually and collectively.

Sleep deprivation is one way the house of medicine systematically depletes the physician's energy. Sleep is vital for physical well-being and plays a pivotal role in emotional trauma recovery, serving as the arena where our brains process and make sense of our experiences. The chronic exhaustion from sleep deprivation zaps our clarity and energy, rendering us less capable of focusing and collaborating to enact systemic changes. Instead, we become trapped in the cycle of day-to-day survival, struggling to find the creative energy required to transform the system.

The Real Price of Doctor Student Loan Debt

I also firmly believe that student loan debt is a powerful deterrent for physicians exerting more agency in the healthcare system. I regularly work with new physicians with a student loan debt of over $500,000. The interest these loans are accruing is staggering. I commonly see two patterns emerge. First, following residency or fellowship (reminder, periods in which they work up to 80 hours *per* week), they continue this breakneck pace, working the same or even more than during training. This inevitably leads to worsening exhaustion, and there is no bandwidth to be involved in groups to do the necessary advocacy work. The crushing debt also leads them to practice scared. They will tolerate incredible abuses by healthcare entities because they feel they have no choice. They literally can't afford to speak up.

The crushing debt, the long hours they're working, compounded by the lack of time for sleep, nurturing relationships, and other human necessities, is like a form of indentured servitude. This is especially appalling when we step back and realize that the profound debt they're repaying to some medical schools includes for-profit schools and non-profit schools with endowments in the millions or billions of dollars. Even more sickening, many are working for healthcare systems raking in huge profits and affording windfalls to board members and shareholders, plus the record profits that insurance companies have made, including during the pandemic—all on the backs of physicians. Remember, we are the profit-generating workhorses of this system. Without us seeing patients, nothing gets billed in our names. The hospital can't function without us—some way to treat your most highly trained, skilled, and profit-generating people within the system.

Rather than relegating us to merely clinical care, we must integrate the perspective and expertise of physicians into healthcare administration. The more leaders and administrators can partner with physicians and see them as valuable healthcare team members, the better. Several healthcare organizations are moving to leadership dyads, in which physicians are paired with administrators or other key leaders to ensure the changes made balance clinical excellence and business considerations.

Building on the last chapter, which introduced the concept of boundaries, boundaries are critical to physicians harnessing their agency. When we say no to extra shifts, that drains us and prevents us from having the time, mental clarity, and energy to do other work that drives change; that is saying yes to channeling our personal and collective agency to be a change agent. Time is our most valuable resource, and we recognize that the system incentives for physicians are generally structured to keep us as worker bees rather than compensating and encouraging us to develop the skills and do the work of being change agents.

Change agents are "anyone with the skill and power to stimulate, facilitate, and coordinate the change effort."[29] A changemaker takes intentional, creative action to solve a societal problem. We desperately need changemakers devoted to upholding the Hippocratic oath and the highest ideals. As Wendy Dean, author of *If I Betray These Words*, says, we need to stand on our square. We know what is ethical and required to provide evidence-based and compassionate care. We know what resources we need to care for patients in a way that we'd expect for ourselves or a family member.

A changemaker takes intentional, creative action to solve a societal problem.[30] The key to recovering from burnout was channeling my caring into effective change-making. When we care and are effective changemakers, we become inspiring advocates. This is a crucial way we reduce burnout in healthcare professionals. The changes need not be huge; even small amounts of agency, as simple as emailing to suggest an improvement to a process in your clinical environment is an act of agency. Combined with the emotional intelligence and compelling narrative, the "changemaking know-how" is how you become an inspiring advocate who transmits positive energy to your team around you.

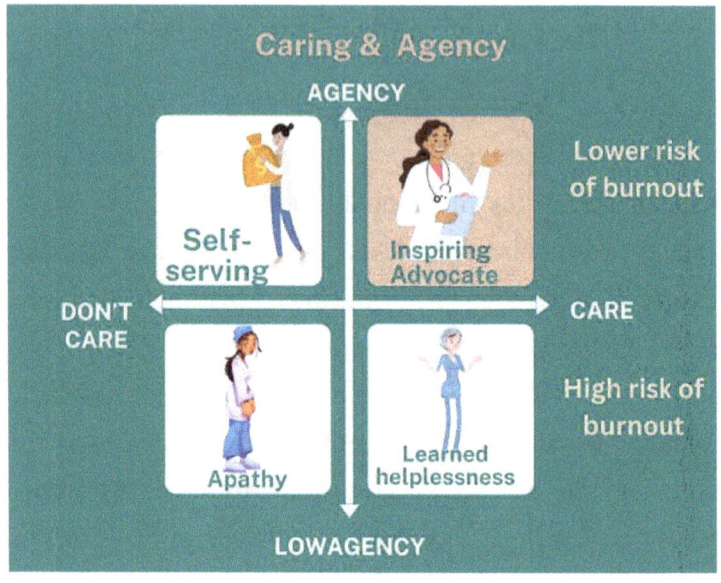

A quadrant chart shows how caring and agency are related. I posit that advocates who harness their agency and show caring in the workplace experience lower burnout. Image credit: Dr. Andrea Austin made with Canva.

As emergency physicians, we are part of the safety net of healthcare. Emergency medicine has prided itself on being the MacGyver of healthcare. We are scrappy, and we figure out how to get a lot done with minimal resources. My question is: How is that working out? The time has come for us to clearly articulate what is required to run a functional emergency department. We must stop enabling a dysfunctional system and start creating changes to build one that works for patients—and doctors.

One tangible example of how we can start doing this is an exciting initiative by the American College of Emergency

Physicians to accredit emergency departments.[31] When we look at trauma centers in the United States, they are accredited by the American College of Surgeons, and there are clear guidelines on what people and resources are required to have a functional trauma center. We urgently need to work towards systems-level solutions to improve healthcare. When thinking about how to do this, in Dr. Verena Voelter's book, *It Takes 5 To Tango*, she outlines an approach to aligning the interests of patients, policymakers, payers, pharma, and providers.

The healthcare system relies heavily on doctors, and without our presence and expertise, it would face significant challenges. In a recent interview with Dr. Leon Adelman, Founder of Ivy Clinicians, he shared that unionization can be a strategy to bring hospitals back to the table to work with physician-owned groups. Hospitals want to avoid unions at all costs - suddenly, working with a group of doctors doesn't seem so bad.

Forming a union is a long process. Depending on how your group is structured, there can be real challenges to creating a union, especially if your group covers multiple hospitals. I'm pro-physician, and unions will be part of this solution. At the same time, we don't have to wait for a union to start being changemakers. We are exceptionally well-trained, highly skilled, and indispensable healthcare team members. We matter; our voices belong at every level, from the bedside to the boardroom.

Reflect:

Think about the concept of agency in your career. How have you exercised personal or collective agency to effect change within your workplace or the broader healthcare context?

Personal agency example:

_____

_____

_____

Collective agency example:

_____

_____

_____

Reframe:

Are there any thought errors in which you minimize your sense of agency? How can you reframe this thought to increase your agency?

_____

_____

_____

Reimagine:

How could your career have more fulfillment, increasing your agency?

_____

_____

_____

Respond:

How can you incorporate the beginner's mindset into your daily practice to renew your passion for healthcare and improve your resilience against burnout?

_____

_____

_____

Resources:

The Persuaders, Part 1 and 2. Brené Brown podcast, _Unlocking Us._

ACEP ED Accreditation. www.acep.org/edap

ACEP Unionization member-developed information paper and resources: www.acep.org/life-as-a-physician/unionization

Dr. Verena Voelter's book, _It Takes 5 To Tango._

Andrea Austin

CHAPTER 14

PARENTING YOURSELF

"There's no one who's going to rescue us if we don't at least do part of that ourselves." —Dr. Christina Shenvi on Heartline podcast, Apr 11, 2023

We each grew up with distinct sets of parents with unique life experiences that shaped their parenting styles. My mother once confided that she had me to have a friend because my father, a deputy sheriff, worked night shifts. Having a child to find a friend encapsulates the root of many challenges I faced in my childhood. These challenges later translated into difficulties in setting boundaries and managing my emotions as I entered adulthood.

During my childhood, I had severely misaligned teeth. Our local dentist presented two potential solutions because my mouth was too small for all my teeth. Braces were a certainty, but he also proposed extracting a few of my permanent teeth to shorten the treatment time and reduce costs. I underwent multiple tooth extractions.

One of these extractions was particularly traumatic. I was only about seven years old. As the dentist forcefully pulled on one of my teeth, I couldn't help but cry. However, instead of offering comfort, the dentist scolded me for my tears and threatened to have my mom leave the room if I didn't stop. My distress reached a point where I began hyperventilating. Finally, the tooth came out, and the dentist casually remarked, "Oh, that's why it hurt so much; there's a third root." Offering no apology, he promptly left the room, leaving me in tears with a bleeding mouth.

It wasn't until I wrote this passage that I fully understood why I have such a strong aversion to anything being placed in my mouth. Several years later, while in the military, I had a rough experience with a dental hygienist. Dental care was mandatory, and I felt compelled to endure the appointment rather than reschedule it. I became upset, which seemed disproportionate to the somewhat rough, although not necessarily abusive, treatment I was receiving. This was a clear example of a trauma response. My reaction wasn't to the present moment of a slightly rough dental cleaning; I was reacting to the unprocessed trauma of my seven-year-old extraction.

Reflecting on that dentist experience from when I was seven, I learned a lasting lesson that has taken nearly three decades to unlearn – the idea that I can't trust my body. He repeatedly invalidated my excruciating pain, insisting that I was wrong and merely being dramatic. Since then, many times, I've endured pain while ignoring my body's signals.

Minimizing the pain of women is increasingly reported as not an exception but a byproduct of a patriarchal and historically misogynistic medical system.[32] The term "hysteria" was the first mental disorder described exclusively in women, dating back to the second millennium BC. It meant "emotional excess" and was a diagnosable condition until 1980 in the DSM-III (considered the diagnostic premier reference for American Psychiatry). Hippocrates reportedly coined the term related to the belief that the disease related to the "hysteron," or uterus. This belief has permeated through medical teaching and has resulted in the othering of women, which has led to disbelief in their pain, especially related to obstetrics and gynecology.[33]

As the recipient of multiple intrauterine devices, IUDs, I have received a paracervical block twice, which was at least an attempt to decrease the discomfort related to the insertion of this device. As a medical student, I watched the placement of several IUDs, which includes "sounding" the uterus, akin to measuring it with a metal rod. As an emergency doctor, I have performed many procedures via procedural sedation, which is the use of medications to provide analgesia and decrease memories related to painful procedures. It is lost on me why we would ram a metal rod into a woman's uterus and not offer sedation. Thankfully, there is a growing movement to believe women and offer sedation and pain medication related to IUD placement.[34]

The IUD can be a superb form of contraception and has other indications for gynecological conditions. Please consult with a trusted healthcare professional regarding your contraceptive options, and I encourage you to seek care from a healthcare provider sensitive to the potential discomfort of any procedure and willing to partner with you regarding the best options for you, including addressing understandable anxiety or pain that may occur with any procedure.

I ultimately never got braces, and my crooked teeth were a source of embarrassment. My current dentist, a kind, gentle woman, shared that the plastic liners available could be an excellent option for straightening my teeth. This also coincided with the pandemic; it was ideal timing with our near-constant mask-wearing in public spaces. I also recognized this as parenting myself. My parents couldn't afford braces, but I could afford the liners now. Instead of holding onto the story of what I didn't get as a child, I could take action to fix my teeth now. In addition, I chose a compassionate, gentle dentist who takes my comfort seriously and understands my anxieties around dental work.

*****

When I first moved to San Diego, I had a cherished possession: a snow globe adorned with a caduceus that had been with me since middle school. This humble snow globe embodied my dedication to studying and achieving my dream of attending medical school. It had been by my side throughout high school, college, and medical school. While it wasn't a pricey item, its value lay in the story it represented.

During my move to San Diego, I remember wrapping it carefully in a trash bag to protect it during the journey. Once I arrived at my new apartment, I placed that bag on the floor. Regrettably, my loving husband inadvertently disposed of it in his bid to tidy up.

For nearly a decade, I thought about that lost snow globe. Then, one day, I had an idea: why not check online to see if I could find another one? A quick eBay search yielded results - I found the exact medical snow globe. While it was slightly more expensive than the original, it cost less than $100. Today, it proudly sits in my office, and every time I pass by it, it makes me smile.

We all carry events that may have left us feeling wronged or hurt. These experiences shape us, but they need not define us. As adults, we can parent ourselves and reclaim agency over our lives.

Reflect:

Consider the concept of "parenting yourself." What areas of your life could benefit from more self-compassion? How might you apply these practices to heal past hurts?

_____

_____

Reimagine:

What could your life look like with this renewed focus on parenting yourself?

_____

_____

Respond:

Consider how you can reconnect with your inner child's joy, curiosity, and wonder. What activities, hobbies, or interests did you love as a child that you've since abandoned? What activity could you add or increase for more joy and fun?

_____

_____

Resource:

Buy Yourself the F*cking Lilies by Tara Schuster

CHAPTER 15

THE ART OF REJUVENATION: CULTIVATING RESTFUL PRACTICES FOR PHYSICIANS

" If you're going to go go go for your whole life, you need to rest and to pay attention to what that rest should look like." — Dr. Leslie Koenig, on the Heartline podcast, Sep 6, 2022

In the autumn of 2023, I participated in a medical fashion show as part of the Women in Medicine Summit™. As part of this event, we each carried signs bearing a message we wanted to convey to the audience. My choice was, "Nevertheless, she thrived." The phrase, "Nevertheless she persisted," gained popularity and was embraced by the feminist movement in 2017. It originated when Senator Mitch McConnell used it as a rebuke to Senator Warren during her passionate objection to the confirmation of Jeff Sessions as Attorney General. The phrase is undeniably a mighty rallying cry. However, I grew weary of mere persistence; I yearned for more – I longed for thriving. I aspire for all women in medicine to thrive, live, and work in alignment with their values, boundaries, and priorities—this vision of thriving challenges the entrenched patriarchal norms within the medical field. To thrive, we must focus on rest.

Rest is a four-letter word in medicine. Medical school is likened to drinking from a firehose. Instead of imparting what's essential, the hidden curriculum insinuates that we should strive to know it all—a fallacy, considering medical knowledge is estimated to double roughly every 73 days.[35] In pursuing this unattainable goal, driven by competition and the desire to outshine our peers, we lose sight of the art of resting. Every moment of our day is transformed into a unit of productivity and, later, as practicing physicians, into an opportunity for generating revenue.

I distinctly recall a moment during my third year of residency while rotating in a bustling emergency department. I paused briefly, trying to gather my thoughts, take a breath, and decide on my next course of action—a moment of rest. Observing my brief reprieve, the attending physician remarked, "What are you doing? There is no rest here. You're always moving, charting; there's no time for rest."

When physicians begin to incorporate rest, we may still gravitate towards motion or something that can be checked off, like reading another book, rather than truly slowing down. During a call with a dear friend, I shared how stressed I was regarding a particular confluence of work and life stressors. She asked, "Andrea, what are you doing for you?" I discussed how I was trying to get back to exercising and listed my various workout strategies. She sighed heavily and said, "That just sounds like more work. I'm talking about rest. Today, I got up and sat outside and looked at the ocean. I didn't read, meditate, or do anything."

The same friend shared a lecture on trauma, and while I was familiar with the trauma responses of fight, flight, fawn, and freeze (also discussed earlier in this book), there were new insights around the flight response. Hyperfunctioning and busyness is a form of flight. I was dumbfounded reading the slide. Yet, it made sense. When we're in constant motion, we don't feel things; we don't stop to consider what we need and what is going on around us. I'm not saying that everyone busy is in a state of flight, but it is worth pondering. What is all that busyness about? I've met countless friends who have returned from difficult deployments and immersed themselves in work again. Several have hit very profound walls years later, me included.

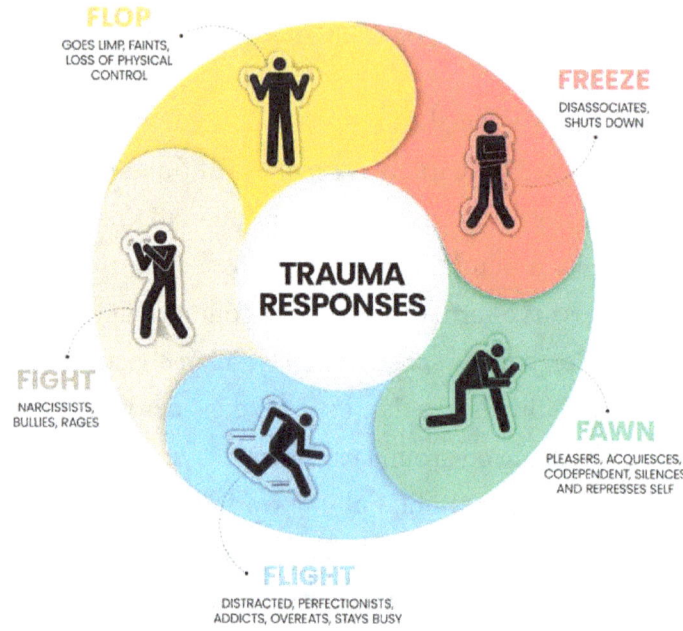

Image credit: Whale Design- stock.adobe.com.

Ironically, incorporating rest into our lives requires some planning. We need different types of rest. *Sacred Rest: Recover Your Life, Renew Your Energy, Restore Your Sanity* by Dr. Saundra Dalton-Smith outlines seven types of rest: physical, mental, emotional, sensory, creative, social, and spiritual.

I am an intellectually curious person. I constantly want to learn, and there are so many books and podcasts out there to support learning. Yet, over the years, I've learned that I can't listen to books or podcasts when driving home from the emergency department. I need mental rest and gravitate towards a playlist of my favorite and familiar songs.

My podcast and much of my work related to medical simulation and writing are creative. Periods of rest are essential to my creativity; overworking zaps it.

As I've aged, sensory rest is also increasingly important. I need quiet after periods of noise, whether from the emergency department, a concert, or a noisy restaurant. This can also be compounded if this noisy environment involves socializing, which is mentally more taxing when in a loud environment.

In the years since my residency, I've started a conscious process of daily rest. Nowadays, I ensure I have a dedicated 30 minutes for rest on most mornings. I make my coffee leisurely, savoring the slow drip brewing process that takes 5-7 minutes. I sit on the couch with my dogs, sipping my coffee deliberately. Usually, I gaze out at my backyard without reading or checking emails, simply being. I can't recall ever doing this during my residency, except perhaps during a vacation. Most days, I hastily devoured a granola bar and dashed out the door. My husband and I had devised a system where, if my car needed gas, we'd swap vehicles to squeeze an extra unit of productivity into my day. Filling up on gas or grocery shopping were luxuries I couldn't afford during those demanding residency years.

How much rest do you require? It's a unique answer for each person, but everyone needs some. If you're new to the idea of rest, aim for at least 15 minutes daily. In my case, rest equals solitude (apart from my dogs). I relish curling up on a couch, preferably with a view. I prefer to be in my home, surrounded by pictures of family and friends, encompassed by greenery. Introducing a couch into my home office was a game-changer, letting me find more moments of rest throughout the day.

How do you recognize when it's time to rest? For me, it's my neck and shoulders that give the signal. When they start tensing up, it's a cue for a mental break and a good stretch. It's also when my thoughts scatter, and I lose clarity and focus. As someone once addicted to productivity, it has taken considerable time to become attuned to these subtle shifts within myself. Medical school and residency instill the ethos of pushing through internal signals. Undoing this conditioning is lengthy and unpredictable, but the rewards of embracing rest are immeasurable.

Many challenges we encounter as physicians cannot be overcome solely through sheer determination. The "grit-only" approach is ingrained in us during medical school. Back then, I often felt devoid of creativity. I also had a narrow understanding of creativity and thought it was for artists, not a valuable trait for physicians to cultivate.

I now understand the immense value of creativity within the field of medicine. We confront many dilemmas— complex issues with no straightforward solutions. Addressing these dilemmas, especially given increasing financial constraints and other emerging challenges, demands more than just grit. Redesigning our healthcare system requires creativity.

Reflect:

Reflect on the quantity and quality of your rest in the seven domains articulated by Dr. Saundra Dalton-Smith:

Physical   Creative

Mental   Social

Emotional   Spiritual

Sensory

_____

_____

_____

Reimagine:

Imagine redesigning your daily routine to include deliberate periods of rest. What activities or moments would you incorporate to ensure you are relaxing and recharging?

_____

_____

Respond:

Given the importance of creativity in addressing complex problems, how can you use your creative thinking in professional dilemmas? Consider adopting new strategies or perspectives that encourage innovative solutions.

_____

_____

_____

Resources:

Dr. Leslie Koenig: Finding the Calm in the Storm. Episode 14, _Heartline_ podcast.

Dr. Leslie Koenig: Going from Reacting to Responding. Episode 15, _Heartline_ podcast.

Sacred Rest: Recover Your Life, Renew Your Energy, Restore Your Sanity by Dr. Saundra Dalton-Smith

CHAPTER 16

MEDITATION

"You can still have that reaction, but meditation helps you notice that reaction quicker." — *Dr. Leslie Koenig, on the Heartline podcast, Sep 6, 2022*

Returning to the formula for revitalization:

Revitalization = Inflection Point + Clarity

How can one reach clarity? Meditation is an effective method for enhancing one's clarity muscles. For individuals in the medical field, meditation might seem contradictory to our profession's high-paced and demanding nature. In this context, sitting still and meditating might seem to be a colossal waste of time.

Yet, my first introduction to meditation was in medical school. There was a mindfulness and meditation program offered as an extracurricular. I was curious but decided I didn't have time for a program like that. It seemed too new age and like a luxury, not a necessity for getting through medicine.

Years later, meditation kept coming up, along with growing scientific evidence it improves brain health and emotional well-being. Meditation is the practice of observing your thoughts. In the initial stages, unless you have innate Yoda-like qualities, what you observe will probably resemble a stream of consciousness—annoying, disorganized, neurotic, and judgmental. It's a shared experience that, for a considerable duration, our thoughts usually meander in various directions. While this might be irksome, there's substantial insight to be gained by understanding the recurring patterns of your thoughts.

My initiation into meditation involved using the Muse™ device, a headband worn across the forehead to detect brain waves. As you meditate, it offers biofeedback through the soothing sound of birds chirping. For those of us with a Type A personality who crave confirmation that we're meditating "correctly," this device serves as a helpful source of positive reinforcement.

Many individuals assert that they cannot or will not engage in meditation, considering the act of doing nothing as a futile use of time. They contend that activities such as walking or swimming serve as their meditation. I, too, have held this belief. However, it's important to differentiate between those for whom walking or swimming is a meditative practice and those who claim it while still trapped in the monkey mind—a frenzied state characterized by a stream of to-do lists and self-criticism. Flow states during exercise can have similar benefits to meditation; consider what your mind is doing during exercise. If your training is focused on hitting specific goals, like distance traveled, calories burned, and weight moved, that may be your focus, and it may be hard to double dip into a flow state, and a meditative state is even less likely.

For those who harbor skepticism about traditional meditation but identify as moving meditators, guided moving meditations offer a potential solution. On days when my body is filled with energy, yet my mind remains agitated, I turn to walking meditation. This practice guides me through a focused awareness, starting with my feet and the sensation of the ground beneath, eventually expanding to include observation of various external stimuli during the walk. It serves as an excellent option for reaping the mindfulness benefits of meditation while expending physical energy.

It's beneficial to distinguish between mindfulness, meditation, and the flow state. Mindfulness practice can be used anytime throughout the day. When I cannot engage in meditation but notice my thoughts spiraling, I am learning to practice mindfulness. I focus on my feet, checking their placement and whether they are in contact with the ground. If there's nervous energy, I might move my toes deliberately and then concentrate on the sensation of my feet on the ground. In a patient encounter, mindfulness involves listening and observing, whether noting details like earrings, how hands are held, or even monitoring lip moisture as an indicator of hydration. There are many ways to infuse mindfulness into every moment. I almost always listen to a patient's lungs during an encounter. Even if it's not "required." I view this as a mindful moment to listen to their breathing, watch the character of the breathing, and focus on attending to them.

Meditation is a deliberate practice of " reeling in our thoughts." Various meditation techniques and observing thoughts increase the potential to change them over time. In my experience, meditation has enabled me to recognize my thoughts more swiftly, view them as passing phenomena, much like boxcars on a train, and decide whether to engage with them or let them pass.

Many doctors gravitate towards flow states, while meditation is less accepted or practiced. Flow is linked to an activity where one becomes immersed, detached from thoughts, and pleasantly "lost" in the task. It is characterized by intense focus and a lack of awareness of time passing. It is a more accessible state for physicians, as in many of our tasks in medicine, for instance, doing a procedure or even writing notes, we can enter flow. During moments of high flow, I can be surprised that several hours have flown by while writing, a significant chunk of time has elapsed in the emergency department, or even an hour has slipped away during a paddling session.

Mindfulness, meditation, and flow each offer unique benefits to our brains. Assess how much of your day, week, or month is dedicated to mindfulness, meditation, and flow periods. Identify what might be hindering more of these moments. Is it the constant lure of social media? There may be an overemphasis on productivity, where downtime feels like an opportunity for work or exercise. Is it a fear of not meditating correctly? Consider noting one to two experiments you could undertake to enhance mindfulness, meditation, or flow in your life.

While the ideal amount of meditation remains a topic of debate, it shouldn't discourage you from starting your meditation journey. In a small study, participants who engaged in 15 minutes of meditation daily after an introductory training day reported similar well-being levels to those on vacation![36] Given that we can't all be on vacation every day, dedicating 15 minutes to meditation is a valuable use of time.[37]

Another common excuse I frequently hear from doctors is, "I'm too busy." Dr. Amishi Jha, during her discussion on Dr. Brené Brown's podcast about her book, "*Peak Mind: Find Your Focus, Own Your Attention, Invest 12 Minutes a Day*," pointed out that caregivers and service-oriented professionals, such as firefighters, experienced a significant improvement in emotional regulation and clarity with just 12 minutes of daily meditation. So, for my Type A, evidence-based friends, there's the minimum we should aim for!

I had the privilege of interviewing Dr. Sheri Dewan, a neurosurgeon, on the *Heartline* podcast. She shared her meditation practice, typically twice daily, for about ten minutes each session. In the morning, her meditation involves visualizing complex surgeries scheduled for the day. This not only helps her rehearse the procedural steps but, more importantly, sets a positive and focused mindset, preparing her for the details of brain surgery. I highlight Dr. Dewan because neurosurgeons are tasked with high-stakes brain and spine surgeries. An error can mean devastating consequences, including loss of speech, paralysis, and death. If someone with such a demanding and high-stakes profession believes in the value of meditation, it speaks volumes.

Reflect:

Reflect on the barriers that have prevented you from practicing meditation or mindfulness. Is it a lack of time, skepticism, or maybe not knowing where to start?

Reimagine:

Visualize yourself engaging in a walking meditation. Where would you choose to walk, and what specific sensations would you focus on during this meditative practice?

_____

_____

_____

Respond:

Identify one small step you can take today to engage in meditation. This could be as simple as a 5-minute breathing exercise or downloading a meditation app. If you have a meditation practice, is there anything you'd like to do to take it to a new level? Maybe a more extended meditation practice or retreat?

_____

_____

_____

Resources:

Take the Impossible and Make it Possible with Dr. Sheri Dewan. Episode 40, _Heartline_ podcast.

Cutting a Path: The Power of Purpose, Discipline, and

Determination by Dr. Sheri Dewan.

Finding Focus and Owning Your Attention interview with Amishi P. Jha. *Dare to Lead* podcast by Brené Brown.

Peak Mind: Find Your Focus, Own Your Attention, Invest 12 Minutes a Day by Amishi P. Jha.

May, C. J., Ostafin, B. D., & Snippe, E. (2020). The relative impact of 15 minutes of meditation compared to a day of vacation in daily life: An exploratory analysis. *The Journal of Positive Psychology*, 15(2), 278–284.

Basso JC, McHale A, Ende V, Oberlin DJ, Suzuki WA. Brief, daily meditation enhances attention, memory, mood, and emotional regulation in non-experienced meditators. Behav Brain Res. 2019 Jan 1;356:208-220.

CHAPTER 17

EMBODIMENT

"When I left for deployment, I joked that I cried all the tears that I had...I don't actually remember crying on deployment at all, despite many times wanting to, but I couldn't get the tears to come. And then when I came home, they didn't really come either." — Dr. Andrea Austin, on Heartline podcast, Nov 15, 2022

Becoming embodied has emerged as a crucial part of my journey toward revitalization. While embodiment is in the zeitgeist, it's not just a passing trend. Embracing embodiment is necessary for the strategies outlined in this book to yield ideal results. As I have said, medical training encourages doctors to become disembodied. I experienced a disconnect from my own body. I became unfamiliar with signals of fatigue and illness. Professionalism is a term used frequently in medicine. This term has been weaponized against doctors, as it is used to guilt or shame us from listening to our bodies. I look forward to a day in medicine when showing up sick is viewed as more unprofessional than lauded as the ultimate sign of professionalism.

Many doctors are people pleasers. Whether this trait was innate or acquired during our medical journey, to a certain degree, people-pleasing becomes necessary for navigating medical school and residency. I recall an attending that oscillated between bubbly and fun, followed by lashing out in very scathing verbal rebukes. I worked so hard to garner her praise and avoid the outbursts. Her moments of praise would feel all the better against the backdrop of a recent tongue-lashing. With rare opportunities to evaluate faculty, trainees too often must endure poor behavior and resort to people-pleasing to survive. We learn to disembody when enduring verbal lashings. We disconnect from hunger, fatigue, muscle pain, and other signals that we are human beings with physical needs.

While disembodiment is harmful to everyone, it is especially detrimental to doctors. Our bodies continually give us signals, and as the supposed experts on human health, how can we effectively teach our patients to interpret their bodily cues when many of us are disembodied?

How can one embrace embodiment? I began with a small but significant step. I established a rule about hydration. If the need arose, and there wasn't an immediate life-threatening situation in the emergency department, I allowed myself to take breaks to ensure my tea mug or water vessel was full and that I drank enough; I had to refill them at least once during my shift. Unlike the dramatic scenarios in medical TV shows, many shifts in the emergency department involve patients with chronic illnesses and sub-acute complaints that should ideally be discussed in a clinic within a functioning healthcare system.

Sometimes, we get caught up in a false sense of urgency. While nobody enjoys waiting, depriving ourselves of fundamental human needs such as using the restroom, eating, and drinking isn't a sustainable approach to a medical career. It's essential to identify or, when necessary, create moments for brief breaks to tend to one's needs.

Addressing hunger was the next step. Despite careful hand hygiene practices on shift, I do not like eating food with my hands. I started packing forkable or spoonable meals that were easy to consume during my shift. Paying attention to hunger and thirst proved crucial, as I experienced less fatigue and irritability by attuning to these needs.

When you visit a massage therapist, they often begin by asking, "Any specific areas you'd like me to focus on?" These areas of concern serve as valuable data points. Personally, my neck and shoulders are always my focal points. As I started my journey toward embodiment, I learned of my tendency to tense and raise my shoulders unconsciously. At first, I wouldn't notice until my neck started hurting, which can lead to tension headaches from prolonged muscle tightening.

Let's return to the body scan exercise introduced in Chapter 5. While there are various approaches to conducting body scans, and for those of us who may feel somewhat disembodied and struggle to detect tension, another method involves trying to tighten the muscles in a specific region before consciously relaxing them. It's revealing when you try to tighten a muscle group only to realize it's already tense from stress. With chronic stress, some muscle groups may not relax instantly.

Despite being on an ongoing journey toward embodiment, I am now more aware of when my muscles are tightening. Instead of powering through, I reflect on the source of tension and ask myself, "What do you need right now?" Many times, the solutions are simple and accessible. Whether it's a brief walk, a few deep breaths, a cup of tea, or a short conversation with a colleague, these actions help relax my body.

Early in medical school, we were instructed that sitting during patient interactions fosters a more comfortable and therapeutic atmosphere. Unfortunately, not all patient care areas are equipped with stools. Absent stools, I used to try to slouch to make myself appear smaller for better eye contact with my patients. However, over time, I realized this was causing neck flares. Nowadays, I try to find a stool or, if none are available, I explain to the patient that I usually sit for this conversation, but stools are unavailable. While it's less than ideal, I avoid slouching to prevent neck strain.

Embodiment is an early warning system for identifying

problematic individuals in your life. Through the practice of embodiment, you become attuned to physical cues like a tightened jaw, stomach discomfort, sweaty palms, or any signals specific to you indicating discomfort around someone. This practice enables you to align with your values and set boundaries effectively. Consider this early warning system as a protective mechanism. When it activates, ask yourself, "What do I need right now?" It might be to exit the situation, seek help, or assert a clear boundary. Instead of ignoring or silencing this early warning signal, you come to appreciate and value it. Through consistent embodiment practice, you may notice how early and subtle these warning signals are, making it easier to address threats or perceived threats at an initial stage.

My journey toward embodiment first involved limited language to express my internal signals. Over time, I've honed my ability to discern and articulate what and where I'm feeling. EMDR therapy has played a significant role in enhancing this skill. During sessions, the therapist prompts, "Where are you feeling (insert emotion) right now?" Through practice, I've developed the capacity to specify, for example, "in my temples" instead of a general "head" and to describe sensations like pulsating.

Being a recovering people pleaser, practicing embodiment is essential for maintaining my integrity. As someone prone to overcommitting, I've learned to recognize the tightness in my chest that signals when my resources are stretched too thin for more projects. Rather than ignoring this sensation, tuning into it lets me uphold my integrity by either declining or responding, "I'll need to think on that and get back to you after reviewing my current obligations."

As you start or continue your journey toward embodiment, I understand the appeal of a checklist! If you find words more comfortable, consider starting with descriptors, making it more straightforward to identify your body cues. Revisiting the PHALLTS mnemonic can guide you: are you in pain, hungry, angry, late, lonely, tired, or stressed? From there, trace back to what may have been the signal in your body, the early warning for this emotion. Where did you feel it in your body? Incorporating a few daily body scans can help you focus on your bodily signals. Following this, you can experiment with strategies to address these signals. For example, if you feel, "I think my eyes are dry. Hmm, that might be because I'm blinking less while on my computer. I'll try using these eye drops and set a timer to remind myself to take a short break every 45 minutes to stretch and blink."

We have opportunities to support each other's embodiment as well. For example, when you observe someone's head bobbing at work due to fatigue, do you overlook it? Or do you shame them by reprimanding them for falling asleep? Could you check in with them? For example, "I noticed you're falling asleep at your computer. What do you need right now? I can cover if you want to take a quick nap." When I've attempted this with my residents, the initial response is almost always, "I'm fine; I can push through."

When they reached an exhausted and overwhelmed state during our debrief, I asked, "Before you hit the wall, what signals were you receiving from your body?" Again, most looked at me as if I'd grown a second head and then replied, "What do you mean?" That exhaustion is rarely a sudden event. Many factors contributed to the exhaustion, and our bodies send us many messages indicating the need for rest before the shutdown phase.

What else hinders embodiment? Numbing out. Many methods exist to dull our bodies and mute the signals they are trying to convey, feeling exhausted. Indulging in a crunchy snack and endless scrolling on social media is a recipe for exhaustion. Screen time and snacking close to bedtime disrupt restorative sleep and reduce our bodies' signals.

I am aware that I experience a specific type of muscle pain with sleep deprivation; it feels distinct from working out at the gym, more intense, and penetrating my muscles. This is a well-documented phenomenon in chronic fatigue syndrome and is also suggested to be a similar process that may induce muscle pain in fibromyalgia. Some trigger points in our body become inflamed or painful with sleep deprivation. How about when we sense this, we engage in restorative activities? Instead of numbing out, we could take a warm bath, use some lavender, avoid screens, and put ourselves to bed.

The inclination to numb out is a conscious or subconscious effort to avoid processing the emotional trauma we encounter in medicine. I've convinced myself that I "need" to watch mindless television to forget or dampen what I've experienced on a shift. However, I now recognize that I must set limits when I feel this pull. Typically, I'll only watch a 30-minute lighthearted show after a shift. If I still sense the magnetic pull of the TV, I ask myself, "Is there something from the shift that I'm trying to numb out right now?" The solution is often to turn off the TV, be still, and see what comes up. I've become so adept at compartmentalizing and disconnecting that it requires a lot of intentionality to realize that a patient interaction needs processing. Especially as I've started processing things sooner and more frequently, the time needed to process and the intensity of the emotions have modulated.

Returning to the opening quote from this chapter, I am still learning to cry again. It's a funny sentence to write, as it implies how much life and trauma change us; something we're hardwired to do becomes stifled. In Stephanie Foo's book *What My Bones Know,* she describes how detaching from oneself can be so insidious. While it may seem obvious that the inability to cry is a form of detachment, it wasn't until I nearly finished writing this book that I saw this in my lack of crying. I lost the ability to cry for years because I had left my body. One of my favorite quotes is from a dear friend, Dr. Christina Shenvi, "We need time to let our soul catch up with our bodies," inspired by a quote from *The Ruthless Elimination of Hurry* by John Mark Comer, in which he states, "The solution to an over-busy life is not more time. It's to slow down and simplify our lives around what really matters."

In the final revision of this book, I had brunch with a dear friend, Dr. Katrina Landa, and she shared slides in a talk she gave on combat stress. Familiar with fight, flight, fawn, and freeze, I read some descriptions beneath each word. Under flight, the descriptors included "anxiety, fear, panic, avoiding, chronic worry, and perfectionism." I sat in a dumbfounded state. I understood the fight response and had my share of irritability and anger over the years. I also understood the fawn response and the people-pleasing and boundary-busting tendencies, but the flight descriptors took my breath away. I never put together that overworking, constant planning, and perfecting were trauma responses and ways to leave my body. They kept me in a left-brain dominant state in which feelings, creativity, play, and rest were not valued. Like a balloon, my brain kept swelling, and slowly but it left my body until one day, it was so far detached that the signals it would try to send, like sadness, couldn't even get my lacrimal ducts to do their designed function.

To this day, a frequent check-in question from my therapist is, "Have you slowed down enough for your soul to catch up with your body?" My frequent reply is, "Working on it, I can at least see my soul now."

I'm not an embodiment guru. There are many books and courses on this subject, and a few are listed below if you want to dig deeper. However, don't let the intellectual pursuit of embodiment hinder your actual state of being embodied. As a doctor, you're accustomed to being in a hyperfunctional, cerebral state. Before adopting this cerebral version, you were born with the innate ability to be embodied. We are intrinsically connected to our bodies, constantly with us. It has evolved to give you ample data at every moment, and every second of the day is an opportunity for you to reconnect and be embodied.

Reflect:

Think about the last time you ignored a basic bodily need (like hunger, thirst, or the need to use the restroom) for productivity or "professionalism." How did it make you feel afterward?

_____

Reimagine:

Envision a form of exercise or movement you genuinely enjoy. Pick one that celebrates what your body can do rather than a punishment or obligation. What activity would that be, and how could you incorporate it more into your life?

_____
_____
_____

Respond:

Choose a bodily need (like hydration, nutrition, or movement) you frequently neglect and commit to addressing it more consciously for one week. Notice any changes in how you feel.

_____
_____

Resources:

How to Follow the Wisdom of Your Body with Dr. Hillary McBride. *We Can Do Hard Things* Ep 206

Practices for Embodied Living and Wisdom of Your Body by Hillary L. McBride.

CHAPTER 18

THERAPEUTIC TRAVEL

"Sometimes, travel gets a bad rap as being frivolous. When done intentionally, I believe travel is integral to our personal development. I am not the same person I would be without the places I've been and the people I've met." — Dr. Andrea Austin

I love exploring new places. However, by the end of February 2022, I was experiencing a familiar sense of exhaustion. Once again, I had ridden another wave of the pandemic. Each wave had its challenges. This one was exacerbating because I was losing track of the waves, and it felt like, as a country, we hadn't done the essential things to decrease transmission or prop up our failing healthcare system. We lost so many experienced staff, and many of those who remained were on their last nerve.

While a beach vacation certainly doesn't serve as an instant remedy for burnout, I've found it a valuable component of my recovery following intense work periods. With only four nights, I knew minimizing travel time and maximizing relaxation was crucial. Kauai, Hawaii, emerged as an excellent choice. My husband, Chris, and I visited Kauai in August 2019, and we explored the island, partaking in recommended activities such as seeing the Napali Coast from the air (via a helicopter tour), sea (on a Catamaran tour) and land (through hiking).

This time, I had a different agenda for my stay at the resort. My plan was simple: indulge in ample sleep, immerse myself in reading and writing, and bask in the sun on the beach. This combination of activities serves as a potent source of restoration for me. It nourishes my mind and offers mental clarity on various personal and professional matters. I've cultivated a routine of retiring to bed at a reasonable hour and rising with the sunrise. This helps me reset my internal body clock, a refreshing change from the jumbled sleep patterns I experience in emergency medicine.

Staying at the same resort was a deliberate decision. The beach was beautiful and not crowded. In addition, there was a bay with calm waters perfect for paddleboarding, one of my cherished water activities. After a splendid day of beachside lounging, I decided to cap off the afternoon with a paddle.

However, something had changed since my last stay at this resort: the paddleboard rental was now on the opposite side of the bay. This side of the bay had slightly higher waves, requiring me to wade out into water that was about waist-deep before hopping onto the board. I've been paddleboarding for over a decade, primarily in San Diego, and ironically, while it's a water-based sport, I typically stay dry. Usually, I would wade out to knee-deep water and effortlessly mount my board. Starting my paddle adventure in a drenched state was humorous. It was amusing to think I was already wet, so falling off my board would be no big deal. Was this my perfectionism creeping into my paddling, and how did it sour my shifts in the emergency department? So much mental energy on shift was on how to "not" not miss a diagnosis, not miss a metric, not get yelled at by a consultant, not disappoint a patient, and not be viewed as lazy by colleagues, which manifests as the first to sign up for a patient, even if I was already feeling overwhelmed. Could I focus on being and doing, rather than the "not," a form of perfectionism and performing, all ploys to avoid shame? Avoiding getting wet was a clear metaphor for all the times my perfectionism prevented the possibility of joy. As I looked out on the horizon, I felt a sacredness coinciding with the somatic experience of paddling. I attuned deeply to this moment in the hope that the cascade of neurons firing loosened the hold of perfectionism on my mind.

As I began my paddleboarding journey, I encountered waves heading my way. I dropped to my knees to maintain balance and avoid tumbling off the board. While the ultimate goal in paddleboarding is to stand, kneeling provides more stability. At first, I felt a tad frustrated by this change. I saw the momentary drop to my knees as a sign of my lack of athleticism and thought that a better paddler could have stayed upright. At the same time, I realized the need for a more compassionate perspective. My usual paddleboarding locale was the serene waters of San Diego Bay. It shouldn't surprise me I needed time to adapt to these more challenging waves. Could I show more self-compassion off my board at work, too?

After reaching the calmer side of the bay, I rose to my feet, smoothly gliding through the water with ease. As I settled into a comfortable rhythm, my thoughts began to drift. Gazing out at the bay, I couldn't help but reflect on the person I was when I last paddled here just under two years ago. Back in 2019, I was still in the Navy, blissfully unaware that I would soon be thrust into the tumultuous challenges of a pandemic as an emergency doctor. This trial would test my physical and mental endurance to the utmost. Yet, as I rode those waves, I recognized that I had undergone a profound transformation, emerging from those trials as a stronger individual.

A few minutes later, another wave approached. I instinctively turned to face it, ready to ride its crest. Paddleboarding taught me that riding a wave is easier when confronting it head-on. Trying to evade it typically results in toppling into the water or, at the very least, being forced down to your knees. This scenario paralleled many of my experiences during the pandemic. I had made concerted efforts to suppress many challenging emotions, particularly my grief and sadness. I kept veering away from these messy emotions when I needed to confront them head-on.

Moments later, the water seemed deceptively calm. I allowed myself to unwind, and my thoughts began to wander again. Suddenly, an unexpected wave crept up on me, nearly causing me to lose my balance and tumble into the water. However, I stayed on the board. It struck me: my body had reacted to the wave before my mind did. My feet instinctively made micro-adjustments, working with my core to keep me upright. It was turning into an oddly reflective paddleboarding session, with the parallels between this day on the board and the tumultuous waves of the pandemic becoming increasingly apparent. My body constantly sends me signals and knows what I need before my mind does. Could I trust my body more and honor what it needs, recognizing the profound wisdom and rapidity of perceptions it has?

As I paddled back to shore, I peered down to gauge whether I was in a shallow enough spot to step off the board. My judgment faltered, and I ended up submerged in the water. Emerging with my hair soaked, I couldn't help but laugh again. Could I hold onto this lighthearted amusement when I returned to the emergency department? Not everything is a laughing matter, but I could approach the less life-and-death challenges with a touch of gentle humor.

***

In the fall of 2022, I started contemplating potential

regrets in life. My mother, who has always been there for me, was growing older, and I reflected on the sacrifices she made during my childhood. Despite our limited financial means, she ensured I had new clothes and dance lessons each year. Later, she even bought me a French horn and private lessons. Yes, she didn't get me braces... but I didn't want for much, despite our lower-middle-class background.

This got me thinking about what I could do to repay her kindness. Knowing her deep pride in her Irish heritage and lifelong dream of traveling abroad, I decided to make her dream come true. So, in the fall of 2022, I picked up the phone and said, "Let's go to Ireland, my treat!"

Fast forward to spring 2023, and we started our journey to Ireland. I was immensely proud of my mother for taking her first international trip and persevering through two canceled flights. I expected a delightful trip filled with Guinness, scenic countryside, and historical insights. However, our tour dug much deeper into Irish history. We learned about the struggles under British rule, the devastating potato famine, and the Irish Revolution. These stories of survival deeply moved me, and I began to view my mother's side of the family as a lineage of survivors. It became clear that their genes carried the weight of generational trauma, and my grandfather's alcohol dependence, which I had once seen as a personal failing, was now framed as a coping mechanism within a much broader narrative that stretched back to Ireland. This journey through Ireland profoundly expanded my compassion for my mom and her family.

Our relationship has grown stronger since I went on this trip with my mother. We talk more frequently. I saw her navigate the challenges of an international trip, and recognizing the personal growth she's achieved since her hospitalization has given me a newfound appreciation for her. Her strength, commitment to managing her health, and dedication to emotional and physical self-care are remarkable.

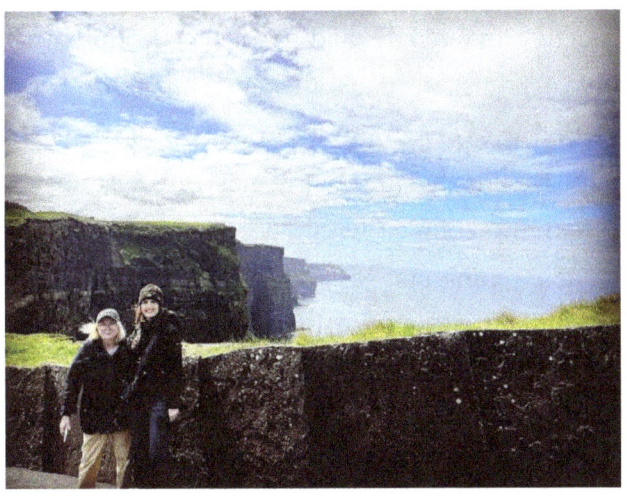

Cliffs of Moher in Ireland with my mom, Mary Austin.

Although I cherished every moment of the trip with my mom, as a self-described ambivert who can swing between extroversion and introversion, I knew I'd require a few days to myself. Before returning to San Diego, I spent time exploring London alone. I indulged in sleeping in, relished eating whatever and whenever I pleased, and strolled around the city at my leisure. One evening, I began my night at the Hotel Savoy with a lavish dinner. Next, I crossed the street to watch Six, a wonderfully entertaining musical about Henry VIII's wives, with a pop music twist and a compelling story of their lives beyond their husband's shadow. While Broadway has its charms, I have a soft spot for London's theater scene.

Many pages of this book came to life in London. The city's energy, the clarity that emerges when inspired by new sights, scents, and people, and the escape from the familiar comforts of home are unparalleled. Although I adore my home, I find it easier to tap into bursts of creativity while traveling. The fresh stimuli my nervous system absorbs during journeys, coupled with the liberation from the daily grind and reminders of various home and work responsibilities, unleash the torrents of creativity that are genuinely exhilarating to ride.

Look at your calendar as you plan your travel for the next few months and years. For example, I have a busy October related to responsibilities to a professional society. Thus, November is an excellent month to plan a restorative trip; some years, that is a beach, and others, it might be a wine trip.

While some of my past trips may have been indulgent escapes, I don't feel like that about my trips now. I seek to cultivate a home life that is enjoyable and sustainable day to day. Every time I fly home to San Diego, I feel like I'm coming home and thankful for the life I've built there. Instead, the travel I pursue now is about expanding from a place of abundance. It's about learning, connecting, and, occasionally, transcendence. Seeing new places, hearing new languages, and eating new foods expands my sense of what is possible.

Reflect:

What type of travel do you crave right now? Is it a trip to an ancestral home to connect with your past? Is it a test of physical strength with an intense hike? Is it a spiritual awakening? A visit to temples, meditation, or yoga retreat?

_____

_____

_____

Reimagine: How could you potentially grow through a therapeutic travel experience?

_____

_____

Respond: What action can you take today to move one step closer to your therapeutic travel trip?

_____

_____

_____

Resources:

Embrace the Wanderlust: How to Thrive as a Digital Nomad Doctor — Dr. Kristine Goins. Episode 55 of _Heartline_ podcast.

Breaking Generational Cycles: Embodiment & Healing Trauma with Prentis Hemphill. _We Can Do Hard Things_ podcast Ep 319.

CHAPTER 19

ADAPTIVE PERFECTIONISM

"Having self-compassion is going to get you a lot farther than berating yourself. Can you imagine how much you could accomplish if you had your own back, and you encouraged yourself? I don't even know what we could accomplish." — Dr. Dinsmore, on Heartline podcast, Jan 9, 2024

I don't know why I am a perfectionist. Looking at my family history, there were none of the classic parenting traits associated with perfectionistic children. While there's a lack of literature about why people become perfectionists, it's sometimes associated with domineering parents exacting standards. My parents weren't like that. In general, they had a laissez-faire style of parenting.

My first memories of perfectionism come from school. Perhaps it was being an only child. I wanted my teachers to like me, and I remember feeling severely uncomfortable with low marks or getting corrected.

In the 5th grade, one of my teachers identified me as a perfectionist. She talked to me one day and referred me to the school guidance counselor to discuss my perfectionism. I remember the first few conversations being pretty awkward. I tried to understand what my teacher and guidance counselor wanted. For me, the point of school was to get high marks, so what did they want me to do? Try less hard?

I don't think my teacher or guidance counselor had the language or at least could break it down for an eleven-year-old. Looking back, they encouraged me to try my best, but as my 5th-grade teacher said, "You're best will do just fine." While I couldn't express myself fully, the phrase felt like a euphuism. It sounded good on an intellectual level, but I didn't feel it in my heart.

After nearly two decades of self-reflection and, later, therapy and coaching, I can provide more language and a road map for perfectionists. A must-read for any perfectionist is *The Perfectionist's Guide to Losing Control* by Katherine Morgan Schafler. The book's thesis contradicts everything I have read on perfectionism and struck a nerve in me. It says there is nothing wrong with being a perfectionist. It defines a perfectionist as someone who sees the difference between the way the world is and how it could be, and they strive for this ideal.

The author eloquently explains that trying to tell someone not to be a perfectionist is the wrong approach. Even worse, it is shaming them about being a perfectionist. Instead, the best approach is to recognize the pitfalls of perfectionism and use an adaptive approach to perfectionism. Looking back on my childhood, the intervention to my perfectionism was rooted in shame: *There's something wrong with you; you need to stop it or suppress your tendency.* While well-intentioned, telling me to say, "Your best will do just fine," didn't explain how to be okay with my best.

Medicine is steeped in practices telling us that our best is not okay. Starting in medical school, comparison and competition are baked into the process. If you don't make AOA (the honor society for medicine), then you will not be able to get into a top residency. If you make a mistake, you will be shamed in Morbidity and Mortality (M&M) process. M&M is a form of peer review, and even to this day, it can be humiliating and shame-inducing. While more people are advocating that to err is human, the malpractice process is such that the reality is that doctors are shamed for errors and face significant consequences that follow throughout their careers.

To navigate perfectionism as doctors, we must do our best and realize that the "best" is highly influenced by many factors, some within our locus of control and others outside our control. Our best also depends on our resources at any given time.

The most important insight was realizing that I needed to decouple my best with the outcome. In some ways, this was taught to me by being a doctor. There are so many cases I can think back on in which we indeed did our best, and the patient ultimately died. While looking for opportunities to learn and grow is essential, overemphasizing every outcome and believing we can control the outcomes is a recipe for disaster. I can do all the right things, and my patient may still die. I can do all the right things and get sued. I can also make a mistake and not get sued. The outcome is not in my control and is affected by factors that aren't fair and don't make sense.

Carol Dweck's book *The Growth Mindset* was one of the most helpful books in my development towards becoming an adaptive perfectionist. She explains that we have two basic tendencies when facing a challenge or setback; one is a fixed mindset in which we think, "I couldn't ever do that," or "I'll always fail when trying." A growth mindset is I still have more to learn, or I didn't get it this time, but I'm committed to trying again. It is helpful to add "yet" to sentences. For example, I haven't hit my mile goal yet. Many people with early achievements, such as in school, can develop fixed mindset tendencies. Then, when placed in more challenging circumstances, they struggle, as they don't have the growth-minded approach that allows them to practice more self-compassion with setbacks.

Along this same line, to quote Dr. Brené Brown, "I'm here to get it right, not be right," is hugely helpful. There are so many things in life and medicine I don't get right the first time. The humility and courage to acknowledge mistakes and make amends are crucial to patients and our healing.

Making amends comes from many traditions. I grew up Catholic, and after confessing a sin, the priest would prescribe an act of service to make amends. For example, if I confessed to talking back to my mom, he may ask that I do an extra chore around the house to make amends. Making amends as a doctor may include reflection and committing to learning more about what contributed to an error, such as attending a course or reading a book. All too often, we don't have mechanisms for amends. Instead, doctors are shamed for any failings or errors, emphasizing punitive rather than restorative ways to keep doctors in the system and growing from mistakes and setbacks.

As a resident, I was involved in a case in which we missed the initial diagnosis, leading to a delay in care. The consultant on the case berated me for the error. Acknowledging what had happened was important to me; I contacted my program leadership and explained the mistake. We agreed that I would present the case at our morbidity and mortality conference. I had the courage to tell my program director what happened because of our culture.

From day one of our M&M introduction, we were told that the focus was on the system's issues contributing to errors and that we would not blame or shame individual physicians. The consultant that was so angry at me initially attended the conference. Following my presentation, she raised her hand. She shared that she felt that the diagnosis was nearly impossible to make initially, that what had resulted was unexpected, and that the care I had rendered was reasonable. This was a healing experience for me, and I'm thankful that this happened during the formative years of my medical education. I now have to remind myself that this is the exception, not the rule currently in medicine. With this in mind, I have to work extra hard to create the conditions with my colleagues to promote a culture where we can share errors and discuss potential solutions.

Being a perfectionist as an emergency physician is particularly draining. The emergency department is far from an ideal place. Nearly every emergency department is crowded. There is a confluence of chaos in our medical system from boarding. This situation results from the lack of inpatient beds, which then causes patients to back up in the emergency department. Other issues include needing more specialists on call to care for certain emergencies, a cumbersome electronic medical record, etc. Expecting perfectionism in this system is laughable, in retrospect. Early on, I expected that I'd never miss a diagnosis, my patients would have a serene experience with minimal waiting, I'd also have idyllic relations with all nurses and support staff, and I'd never get yelled at or have a tense moment with a consultant. I've never had a perfect shift. Every shift, someone is unhappy. In most shifts, many people are disappointed, between patients waiting to be seen or admitted and consultants being woken up during the night to my phone call. In these moments, recognizing what is in my control and what is out of it is helpful. I can't control the consultant being upset that I've woken them. I also don't need to internalize every piece of feedback; for example, their reaction to being awakened likely has far more to do with their tiredness than my medical knowledge.

Katherine Morgan Schafler describes one flavor of perfectionism called the Parisian Perfectionist. This archetype is focused on perfect relationships. They want harmony at all times and work very hard to twist themselves into all sorts of contortions to keep the peace. I recognize this tendency in me and that it results from a desire to buffer situations. I can increase my discomfort to ensure they are more comfortable. Now, I am much more comfortable with people being unhappy, annoyed, irritated, or other negative emotions, and I don't always rush in to soothe them. One of the most powerful ways to stop people pleasing is to develop a mantra, "Let people be wrong about you." This is a radical idea for well-practiced people pleasers. We falsely believe that if we contort ourselves sufficiently, we can control what people think about us! This is a powerful and draining thought distortion. You cannot control anyone's thoughts about you. Sometimes, people will unload on you, and it frequently has nothing to do with you. You were a nearby and sometimes the easiest target.

People unloading on you frequently or particularly blisteringly may be emotionally immature adults (EIAs). Learning about EIAs changed my life. I first heard the term on Glennon Doyle's podcast. Her guest, Lindsay C. Gibson, outlines how people can become psychologically stunted, and this severely affects the way they interact with people.[38] A tell-tale sign is when you're talking with someone, and while you're being calm and logical, suddenly they go on the attack. The attack may be insults or guilt trips—the approach varies, resulting in "brain scramble," the feeling you get when speaking to an EIA, as you're confused about why the conversation has taken this weird, aggressive tone. My therapist recommends that when you've recognized that you're speaking with an EIA, imagine talking to them at the age at which they are acting. Often, this may be someone in middle or high school; sometimes, people regress to a full-on toddler tantrum. In these cases, speaking to them compassionately but not condescendingly is critical. At the same time, don't forsake yourself and your boundaries.

Dr. Brené Brown's research shows that the most compassionate people practice the most boundaries. I can only give from a full cup. This means that if I don't have what I need to console or soothe someone, instead of overextending myself, the best thing for everyone is to step back and do what is required to return to a more compassionate place.

Understanding how compassion and boundaries intersect in healthcare is vital to crafting a fulfilling career. Most healthcare professionals have high levels of compassion. The problem is that many of us did not develop healthy boundaries due to family dynamics and societal expectations, especially for those who belong to marginalized groups. Later, in medical school, many of us entered a system that rewards low boundaries and high people-pleasing or bleeding heart-type behaviors.

Healthcare is a service industry. Healthcare professionals should be fairly compensated. Yet, this field requires compassion. There is an emerging body of literature that patients perceive compassion, which likely impacts their healing. Boundaries without compassion and awareness for our patients and colleagues' feelings can cross over into self-serving behavior… and don't make for great interactions. I doubt self-serving people made it this far in the book… but I bring it up because, as leaders, we need to recognize self-serving behavior.

I've watched colleagues with a leadership title routinely show up late, leave early, and not pull their fair share on shifts. They are holding the boundaries around their time…yet they are not being compassionate or considerate about the impact of their behavior on colleagues. As true leaders, we need to recognize self-serving behavior and dare to call it out and hold people accountable.

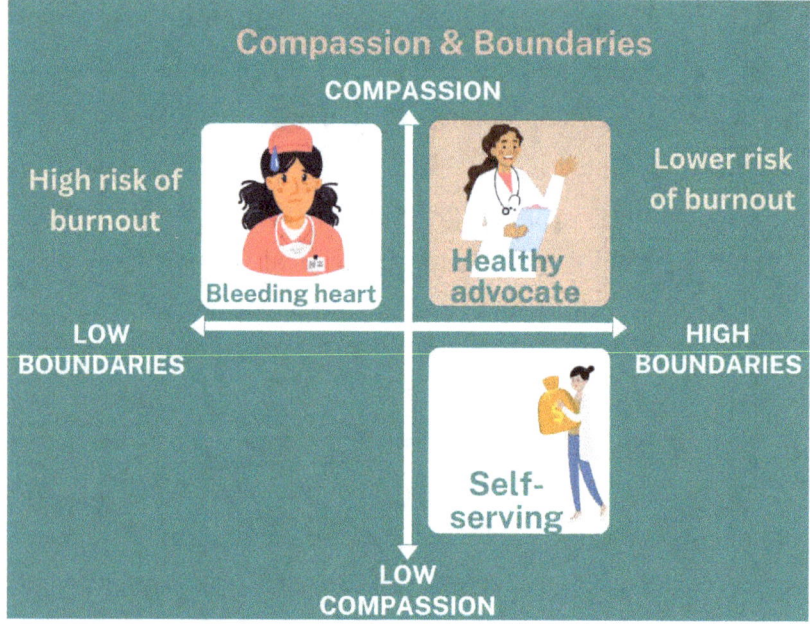

Matrix of compassion vs. boundaries: The goal is to be a healthy advocate for our patients with high compassion and boundaries. Image credit: Dr. Andrea Austin made with Canva.

The key to getting to this place was believing that I was worthy. I am worthy even when people are upset at me. I can feel guilty but avoid the shame spiral. Dr. Brené Brown's work differentiates guilt, as "I did something bad (or not ideal)," from shame, "I am bad." We are worthy even when we mess up.

Based on Dr. Brown's work, the path to staying out of

the shame spiral includes connection. This occurs when we reach out and appropriately and safely share what is going on with a trusted confidant. In addition, when appropriate, extend the amends. Note that the amends doesn't always mean, "I'm sorry." Sometimes, it's inappropriate or unsafe to apologize to someone, or even possible. Even a pause to reflect and think about how to handle a situation differently in the future is an act of amends.

Returning to shame, I now recognize that a maladaptive strategy I developed was shame avoidance. In the emergency department, many metrics related to physician performance are tracked. One set of metrics that causes a lot of angst in the physician community is sepsis metrics. Like most metrics, they start with good intentions. The idea is that we identify sepsis, a potentially life-threatening infection, quickly, start antibiotics and monitor specific lab markers carefully as we resuscitate the patient.

Emergency medicine involves many turnovers, in which the off-going colleague "turns over" their current cases to the oncoming doctor. One afternoon, one of my ER friends turned over a patient with an elevated lactate level. Lactate levels can be elevated for many reasons, including sepsis. The challenge for emergency doctors is that patients usually come in undifferentiated, which means we don't know what's wrong with them. The problem with sepsis is we know that delays in antibiotics can be associated with an increased risk of mortality. As my friend turned the patient over, she relayed that she didn't think it was sepsis and would document that in her note. Charts with an elevated lactate are automatically reviewed, and my shame avoidance kicked into high gear. I went on a soliloquy about how I would not get "flagged" on this chart. As a perfectionist, getting an email or text message from the nurse who reviews the charts and being told I missed or delayed something, even when not true, was like getting an F.

To avoid the shame avoidance spiral, I turn to a tried-and-true technique in these situations: what is best for the patient? Even with all our medical science, there is still a lot of uncertainty around diagnosis and management, especially in the emergency department. With this in mind, I have to give myself the grace to do my best to get it right, not be right (thanks, Dr. Brené Brown again), for my patients—no metric accounts for this complexity.

The following day, I called my friend and apologized for my less-than-collegial turnover. We had a great conversation and acknowledged how thankful we were that we were committed to doing the work to keep growing, learning, and expressing vulnerability. For me, that was confiding that I am a perfectionist, and shame avoidance is a familiar and comfortable place for me to go. This is a beautiful example of the sentiment shared by Prentis Hemphill in an episode of *We Can Do Hard Things:*

"…doing my work helped me do my work in the world."[39] This quote is beautiful because doing the work, having these hard conversations, and allowing for the repair after the rupture lets us keep doing the work of doctoring. When we let moments go by, don't have vulnerable conversations, or don't allow for the potential of deeper understanding and healing, it makes doing the work of doctoring harder. Yes, the work is hard, but not doing the work is more arduous in the long term.

In the emergency department, we have to switch between extremes, from the death of a patient to interacting with someone with a minor complaint, such as an ankle sprain. Switching gears is sometimes tricky, and I've developed practices to help me switch gears and ensure I can show up effectively with the ankle sprain. Note I said "effectively," not "perfectly." I know that I may need to walk outside, take three sips of tea, and pray for the serenity to return to the rest of my shift and that, meanwhile, the person waiting for me is possibly getting more annoyed due to the delay. I am genuinely sorry for the delays, as I also despise waiting for things. Yet, I know that being the Parisian Perfectionist is not sustainable. If I had kept on that path, I wouldn't have been able to do this job much longer.

Learning that my brain will always see that gap between reality and the ideal, yet I have the choice of how and when I engage in closing this gap, was liberating. I love the perfectionist inside of me. I give her a name and recognize when she rears her head. But I am the CEO of my life, and I can tell her to pipe down sometimes.

Reflect:

Are there any areas in your life that show maladaptive perfectionism? What are some of the frequent triggers of your perfectionism?

_____

_____

_____

Reimagine:

What would your life look like if you had more self-compassion and moved from maladaptive to adaptive perfectionism?

_____

_____

_____

Respond:

What is one action you want to take to practice more adaptive perfectionism? From this chapter, some ideas include developing a mantra, seeking therapy, reframing thoughts, and talking to yourself like a friend in challenging moments.

_____

_____

_____

Resources:

The Perfectionist's Guide to Losing Control by Katherine Morgan Schafler

*The Growth Mindse*t by Carol Dweck

The Gifts of Imperfection by Brené Brown is one of the most beautiful books I return to often.

Andrea Austin

CHAPTER 20

PARTNERING WELL

"I've been out of the dating game a long time. My only advice is that if you're hustling for love, you better hustle right on out of that relationship." — Dr. Andrea Austin, Love While Doctoring, published February 14, 2024

Following my divorce in medical school, I told myself I would never get married again. Yet, within a few years, I fell in love with my current husband, Chris. When I left my first marriage, I developed a long list of things I would not tolerate in a relationship. While I didn't have the word boundaries in my vocabulary, effectively, I had developed critical boundaries that would keep me safe and future relationships healthy.

Chris is not perfect. Sometimes, when looking for a partner, we get caught up in finding the ideal person. The key to our marriage has been growing. We are far from the same people we were when we met. We navigate each other's changing interests and needs.

The Gottmans are two married relationship experts who discuss the four horsemen of divorce: contempt, criticism, defensiveness, and stonewalling.[40] Early in our marriage, as a leftover from my previous relationship, I sometimes yelled and was unfair during disagreements. Looking back on my childhood, I didn't have a ton of modeling on different ways to express myself when sad, frustrated, or angry. It took time (and therapy) first to feel my feelings. I had to learn to understand my body's warning signals.

Chris is an engineer, and as of now, I make more money than him. After the experience with my ex-husband ("What does it matter, you're going to be a doctor anyway?"), I felt uneasy about whether Chris was attracted to me or my earning potential. When working long hours, I would say, "You'd be better off with someone with a better schedule. You shouldn't be with me. Look how much time you have to spend on your own." Finally, one day, he said, "You have to stop saying that. I want to be with you. If you keep saying that, it will end us."

Looking back, I was scared of getting hurt. My insecurity manifested as these attempts to "test" him with these phrases. The comments I made to him were an attempt at self-sabotage; I wasn't sure I was worthy of being with Chris, so I was throwing emotional flames at the relationship. Thankfully, he set down this boundary that helped our relationship.

I want to keep talking about money because this is an essential topic for women professionals. When we were first married, I kept my checking account, and Chris couldn't access that account. My paychecks went into this account, and I deposited money into a joint account for joint expenses. Over the years, this has morphed, and we have much more intertwined finances. I appreciate Chris's patience that even once married, I needed the space to keep my autonomy, including financially.

While this may not be true for all relationships, having a lot of overlap in our personalities and interests helps Chris and me tremendously. We are both intense people, voracious readers, fast-paced and enjoy challenges. We also have similar aesthetic taste, which makes tailoring our home and making big purchases much more straightforward.

Anyone who looks at my husband will think he is a "man's man." He is tall, strong, and athletic. He is also very comfortable in his masculinity and doesn't shy away from what has been typically associated with "women's work" in our society. He cooks, bakes, and loves decorating our house for various holidays. His podcasts and reading list include books on women's experiences, strengthening our bond and his capacity to understand my experience as a woman in medicine and our society.

Another lesson I've learned is that you can love someone and not like them. I loved my first husband. I've loved a few other men and realized that love alone is not enough. I like Chris. He's fun to hang out with. I love talking to him on the phone; he is my favorite trip companion. Life is better with him.

I've been out of the dating game a long time. My only advice is that if you're hustling for love, you better hustle out of that relationship. Chris and I never played games. It was never the will he, won't he, call me, text me back dynamic. Thinking back to when that happened in other relationships made my stomach turn. I always felt like we were on equal footing and that I wasn't waiting to be picked or selected, but a mutual understanding, and we both liked and respected each other and later loved each other.

A common phrase in our culture is that marriage takes work. Chris and I sheepishly smile at each other when someone utters these words. We're going on eleven years married, thirteen years together, and there's never been a day that's felt like work. I appreciate that some marriages require more work than others, but the work shouldn't involve you contorting to be another version of yourself. We can all grow, but make sure that growth is along the heartline, to your true essence.

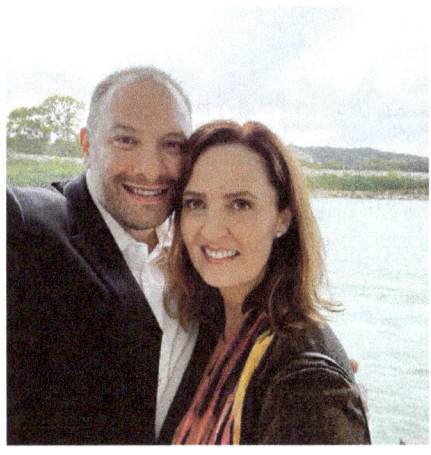

Chris and me in France in October of 2022, celebrating our tenth anniversary.

Reflect:

Sometimes boundaries get crossed or not even established in a relationship. Are there some boundaries you need to re-negotiate?

_____

_____

Reimagine:

Consider new possibilities for greater connection. How would your life look if you improved your current relationships or created new connections?

_____

_____

Respond:

Choose an action to strengthen the quality or quantity of connections. It may be creating or communicating a new boundary, having a tough conversation, or protecting more time to nurture and grow connections.

_____

_____

Resources:

On Love and Divorce while Doctoring. *Heartline* podcast. Episode 26.

Unlocking Us with Brené Brown: Dr. John Gottman and Dr. Julie Gottman on *What Makes Love Last*. February 3, 2021.

The Four Horsemen: The Antidotes. The Gottman Institute. https://www.gottman.com/blog/the-four-horsemen-the-antidotes/

Should Doctors Get a Pre-Nup? April 21, 2023. https://helloprenup.com/prenuptial-agreements/should-doctors-get-a-prenup/

Robert S. Hoffman and Jennie Smith. Physicians: When Do You Need A Postnuptial Agreement? https://mdmonthly.com/physicians-need-postnuptial-agreement/

CHAPTER 21

AUTHENTIC NETWORKING

"If you can have a network of those people in your life who are friends and mentors who raise your game, then it's very important. And for me, I think it's become really essential." —
Dr. Cheryl Martin on Heartline podcast, January 30, 2024

Networking is often a phrase that causes women, especially, to recoil. It usually brings up images of men playing golf or grabbing drinks after work, to this day, spaces that are sometimes off-limits to women. I don't know where I got the networking bug. It may be traced back to growing up in Iowa and not feeling like I had access to the right group of people who could help me get to where I was going. This propelled me to write that first letter to Dr. Mahone to shadow her, which helped me get the letter of recommendation to go to medical school.

I don't use the word networking much anymore. I much prefer the term connecting. Connecting is about building relationships. Strengthening and diversifying these relationships enriches my life and helps me have many sources of support when challenges arise. As my connections grow, I can also connect with others. Connecting a colleague with someone else who can help them grow brings me great joy.

The research on networking has shown that weak ties are an essential and often overlooked networking area. Moderately weak ties, like acquaintances rather than our close colleagues or friends, are the most helpful in finding a job.[41] In the virtual era, weak ties include connections through social media. This has been my lived experience as well. I learned about my simulation director position from a resident who messaged me via Twitter (now X). Likewise, the opportunities to present or get more involved in my professional society often result from those I know less well than my current workplace's tight network.

Networks are also a way to increase exposure to diversity of thought. For example, I belong to the Recalibrate© alumni, a group of physicians who have completed an immersive development program for physicians. Many graduates live in Australia and New Zealand, exposing me to how they practice and approach medicine. I'm active in the American College of Emergency Physicians, which connects me to leaders nationwide and helps me gain different perspectives on approaching our specialty's many challenges.

"Your network is your net worth." - Porter Gale

In the current state of healthcare, overly investing in our current employer's network can leave us vulnerable if we lose that position. For example, who do you turn to if all your mentors, sponsors, and peer mentors are inside that organization and you leave? Your expansive and varied network makes you better positioned to bounce back from setbacks. A diverse network can also expose you to ideas and trends earlier, helping you to position yourself better for the changing tides in healthcare. For example, one of my professors in my master's program has included me in papers on artificial intelligence, positioning me to be a leader in the smart integration of this emerging technology.

How do you get started with networking? It can feel awkward and daunting at first. Authenticity while networking is essential. No one likes someone that feels fake. The best strategy is to network from a place of curiosity. I'm inherently curious about people. Usually, the conversation will flow by starting with basic questions, such as where they live and what they do. Attending a networking reception is helpful when there is a prompt to start the conversation. If the networking reception is about diversified careers, my name tag would say, "Ask me about podcasting" or "Ask me about medical simulation."

Social media can also be a powerful way of connecting. During the pandemic, Dr. Mark Shapiro started a hashtag called #MedLasso. He added to posts about how the hit Apple TV show, Ted Lasso, connects to medical leadership and culture. Adding this hashtag, I connected with Dr. Cheryl Martin, an emergency medicine physician, and *The*

Mind Full Medic podcast host. Cheryl and I soon learned that we shared many interests and began amplifying via social media by re-posting and commenting on each other's work. When I contracted COVID-19 (a mild case), she sent me a gift box full of thoughtful items, including hot cocoa and books, to nurse me back to health. Later, she visited me in San Diego, which was delightful, strengthening our bond as friends and collaborators. Cheryl has subsequently connected me with many doctors and thought leaders in the well-being space globally, as her network includes Australia, New Zealand, and the United Kingdom.

Social media can be time-consuming, and there is increasing evidence it can also have severe negative impacts on our emotional well-being. To get the best of social media, I recommend placing limits on how much time you spend on it. There are settings or apps you can download that will track your time on social media, and you can create limits in which the social media app will not open after you reach a determined amount of time—in addition, avoiding comparisons while on social media is also essential. Sometimes, you can get discouraged by seeing how many friends/followers someone has or that their post went viral and has thousands of likes or re-posts. First, you don't need that many followers or "likes" for your network to pay dividends. At the same time, there are many strategies for social media, recognizing that quality interactions over quantity can be a successful and less stressful way. In addition, remember that your comparisons may not be on the same level, meaning that some people with huge followings have a team supporting their social media presence. For example, they may have a public relations firm or other support that helps them with content planning, posting, and growing their followers. Last, I like using Glennon Doyle's "Block and Bless" strategy to decrease negativity in my social media feed. Recognize that you don't have to accept every request and that there are many predatory people (or bots) on social media.

Mostly, I've had a circuitous approach to networking— no clear plan on who I'll interact with at any event or meeting. While no longer recoiling at networking, having a plan for networking at first glance seemed opportunistic. Now, I've shifted my thought on this, thanks to Scott Galloway, whom I heard on the podcast *Pivot*. His networking tip was to list people you intend to seek during a conference. It's a strategic way to connect with people, recognizing that time is a precious resource. It's about being intentional and in tune with your goals. There's a tactful way to approach seeking people out, especially high-profile and busy people. Yet, most of these people are open to a brief conversation, and more than you'd expect, they are genuinely interested in you and your ideas. As for networking, like so much in life, you'll miss 100% of the connections you don't seek.

"My Golden Rule of Networking is simple: Don't keep score."– Harvey Mackay

I also believe deeply in the karma of networking. I have been so blessed by the doors opened by more experienced and established people in my field. I go out of my way to assist students that contact me. I can't always provide everything they want or need, but I do my best to link them with the resources, entity, or person if I can't address their request. I hope that modeling this behavior inspires them to do more of the same when they're more senior. However, the balance is understanding your limitations and ensuring you only give from a place of abundance. If you're unable to help or get back to someone in a reasonable time window, at least reply to that effect. Pro tip: If you are a person that others regularly seek advice from, and you have the same conversation or send the same email, harness your wisdom. It may be a draft email you can personalize, a blog article, or a podcast episode; you get the idea. I will forward a blog article on how to get started in your simulation career and then have a follow-up conversation with someone so it can be a more personalized and valuable conversation than what was in the article.

Lastly, cards can also be a way to strengthen ties in your network. I keep a file folder with birthday, sympathy, get well, thinking of you, thank you, congratulations, and blank cards. I love cards, but it's tough to find the time to shop for cards for one-off occasions. On a trip to London, I visited the famous department store Harrods and found some fantastic cards. In this digital age, a handwritten card can form a memorable connection. Like everything in this book, don't be phony and only pour from a full cup. Send cards from your heartline.

How to get started with growing your connections:

Reflect:

What career area would you like to grow in, and do you feel networking will be vital to that development?

_____

_____

_____

Reimagine:

How might you connect with more like-minded individuals active in that area? Consider social media platforms, hashtags, and how to friend/connect with these individuals. Are there conferences that attract this group? Conferences are a great way to connect and grow your network, as the in-person energy and spontaneous conversations can be beneficial.

_____

Respond:

Identify 1-2 weak ties with whom you'd like to connect virtually or at an upcoming in-person event.

After connecting with them virtually or in person, note how to follow up with them. This could include a short email thanking them or a virtual meeting.

_____

_____

_____

Resources:

The Frentor Effect: How Peer Coaching Creates Healthcare Synergy with Dr. Cheryl Martin. *Heartline* podcast. Episode 63.

Check out the wonderful podcasts mentioned in this chapter:

The Mind Full Medic Podcast by Dr. Cheryl Martin.

Explore the Space Podcast by Dr. Mark Shapiro

CHAPTER 22

BUILD YOUR BOARD OF DIRECTORS

"The world is becoming more global, and we need to continue connecting with and learning from people from all different backgrounds." — Dr. Sheri Dewan, on Heartline podcast, Jul 5, 2023

A board of directors generally comprises stakeholders with various areas of expertise that advise the Chair, President, or CEO of an organization. I want you to visualize yourself as the CEO of your life. It's your life. You can decide how you live it, yet wisdom and diversity of thought are beneficial. Unlike some boards, this one can't overrule you and force you into doing anything you don't want to do. In the end (the best and worst part of adulting), you have to decide. Figuring out how to leverage the members of your board of directors in your life to get the best advice (and deviate from their advice) is the journey of a lifetime. As a start, though, learning about the types of advisors can help you form your team and be aware of their limitations.

There is no Yoda with a clear path to enlightenment and fulfillment for any of us. There is an over-emphasis on the value of mentors and an undervaluing of people's other roles in our professional development. I want to highlight the definitions of various terms and then unpack how to use the different types of support correctly.

Advisor

This person may have an official role in a school or residency program where they perform specific functions to ensure your successful completion, such as ensuring you're registered for the correct courses to complete graduation requirements. They may have little overlap with your career aspirations, so a trap can be expecting your advisor to fulfill one or more responsibilities of the later described terms.

Mentor

A mentor is more experienced than you and offers advice on one or more aspects of your career or life. The most common mistake I see with mentors is expecting this person to be the Yoda of your career, that they will know what is truly in your best interest, that they alone can open every door you need, and that they are always correct on everything. Most of our careers are complex; thus, we'll need various mentors with different expertise and strengths simultaneously to succeed. In addition, there will never be one mentor who aligns with your values and priorities or has had the same experiences as you. Understanding these limitations helps you know what a mentor can and cannot offer you and will help you avoid the trap of hanging too much on their advice. If you have people-pleasing tendencies, you are particularly susceptible to overreliance on a mentor's input, as you may treat them more like a parent or figurehead who deserves pleasing or obeying. Also, if you have a mentor being paternalistic and overly prescriptive… remove yourself from that relationship.

Frentor

This is a term I've coined for a person who is part friend and mentor. Like a mentor, this person is more experienced and someone you seek advice. Unlike a professional mentor, you share more information about your personal life (commiserate with the friend level) and have a more casual and friend-like dynamic. As a woman physician, I've found frentors critical in my personal development. These women I've felt a special connection with and get along with as friends, yet they also are farther along in their careers and can advise me in a mentor-like fashion. Frentors are especially helpful when something is going on in your personal life, as they can help you navigate the potential implications and strategies to navigate the challenge professionally—for example, decisions about your professional load while being a new mom. The key to a frentor relationship is trust. Sharing information about your personal life, such as considering pregnancy, navigating marital problems, or a personal health issue, is inherently sensitive and can have profound professional implications. There must be a high level of trust to divulge the personal aspects of our lives. While one could argue you could get this support from your friends or a therapist, it's different. Having frentors, people who are more experienced in a domain and have some critical insights into the contextual factors of your personal life, can be crucial in navigating a career.

Peer mentor

If you are someone of a similar rank or position, you can support each other's professional development together. Work in the modern era is complex. It's impossible to have expertise in everything. Even if you're on the same level as someone at work, they have different strengths than you. For example, one of my peers is excellent at leveraging technology for project management. I've been able to share how we can improve the quality of our simulations. While it doesn't need to be a one-for-one trade, you want to reciprocate as a peer mentor, which may be as simple as speaking up to support them during a staff meeting or sharing their accomplishment with the group via email.

Sponsor

While mentors serve a vital purpose, a sponsor takes the additional step of opening doors by taking steps to create opportunities. After I returned home from deployment, I was up for a new set of orders (job) in the Navy. My heart was set on the competitive position at the Navy Trauma Training

Center (NTTC) I discussed earlier in the book. The founder of NTTC, Dr. Kerry King, went out of his way to sponsor me. He made a few calls on my behalf, describing my unique blend of simulation education and military medicine experience. A sponsor takes a risk and spends some of their social capital on the individual they are sponsoring. While mentoring gets much of the focus for women in medicine, some studies show we are over-mentored and under-sponsored.[42]

A sponsor goes beyond the role of a traditional mentor by seeking opportunities and leveraging their social capital on your development. For example, a sponsor may recommend you for a new position. Sponsors have full plates and vast networks. The sponsor may lighten their load by suggesting you take the lead on a project, be the first author on a paper, or other high visibility position. They are staking part of their reputation on your behalf. Seek out sponsors and share your goals. Look for ways to align with them, help them lighten their load, and advance your ultimate goals.

Ally

This is someone who provides support. In the social justice movement, an ally extends this support to someone belonging to a marginalized group. I've had many powerful allies in my career, and I pay this forward by being an ally to others. It's crucial to cultivate allies to keep your well-being cup full. It helps to lean on others to speak up and advocate for you; when your cup is full, you can do this for others as well.

Accomplice

This is a term also used in social justice for someone who goes beyond allyship and seeks to dismantle systems of oppression. Accomplices are key, as there is so much injustice. Especially if you are drawn to getting involved in larger change efforts, building your team of accomplices is important to be more effective and keep your well-being cup full.

In addition to these professional forms of support, you need other advisors on your board. A partner is on your board if you're in a serious relationship. If you don't want your partner on the board, that is a sign that you must reevaluate that relationship. Parents may be on the board, or at least for a while in your career. For some, parents may always occupy a seat, although, for most, their stake on the board becomes less as you mature. Siblings and other family may also have a seat. When healthy boundaries are maintained, family can provide a historical perspective and remind you of your values and inherent gifts (recognizing this is far from the case for some people). It is also alright if your family has been removed from your board.

For me, friends are also on the board—not every friend,

but those in your inner circle. One of my friends and I use a phrase: "This is going in the vault." Things in the vault are not to be shared. The friends who know what is in the vault are well-positioned to advise you on various aspects of your life and have the insight to understand what you should avoid.

Your board of directors may include a therapist, coach, or spiritual advisor. Depending on your life situation, you may also need to expand your board to include a physician if navigating a particularly profound health situation. Lawyers, financial advisors, and other people with specialized expertise or insights may also be on your board or at least stop by to give advice.

Do not confound advice with a directive. When I was younger, it was alluring to follow the advice of mentors mindlessly. In one situation, this led to a professional misstep. My boss assigned me to a military mentor to "enhance my military bearing." While initially reticent, I found the mentor to be engaging and supportive. She advised me to forward my idea of increasing the use of simulation at our command to a senior leader. I asked a couple of times about starting with my supervisor, and she assured me that because it was about simulation, it was okay to go directly to the person who could increase the resources. Predictably, my program director was disappointed that I did not bring the idea to her first. My idea, while great, died. While somewhat painful, this experience taught me it doesn't matter the titles and expertise of anyone on your board of directors. While your intuition isn't always correct, it signals you should at least explore whenever possible before deciding. Sometimes, someone on your board fires off advice without knowing the full context of your life. Remember, only you have the whole perspective of your life and how a decision will potentially impact it. Part of living courageously is following your needs and desires. It is very tempting to defer the decision to someone you hold on a pedestal. Know that when you do this, you're risking your integrity. Slow down, breathe, and follow your heartline to make the tough calls.

Reflect:

Think about the individuals who have significantly influenced your career and personal growth. What qualities did they have that made their guidance valuable to you?

_____

_____

_____

Reimagine:

Imagine your ideal Personal Board of Directors. Who would be on it, and why?

_____

_____

_____

Respond:

List three actionable steps you can take this week to connect with or contact potential Personal Board of Directors members. How will you start these conversations, and what specific topics or areas of guidance will you seek from them?

_____

_____

_____

Resources:

Take the Impossible and Make it Possible with Dr. Sheri Dewan. *Heartline* podcast. Episode 40.

The Frentor Effect: How Peer Coaching Creates Healthcare Synergy with Dr. Cheryl Martin. *Heartline* podcast. Episode 63.

Want to Advance in Your Career? Build Your Own Board of Directors by Susan Stelter. *Harvard Business Review.* May 09, 2022

Ally or Accomplice? The Language of Activism by Colleen Clemens.   www.learningforjustice.org/magazine/ally-or-accomplice-the-language-of-activism. June 5, 2017.

CHAPTER 23

GROUNDED GRATITUDE

"Embrace authentic moments of gratitude, such as thanking someone who helped you during a particularly stressful day. You're not thankful that the day was a dumpster fire, but you can be thankful for the people that made it a bit more tolerable." — Dr. Andrea Austin, *Top Revitalizations of 2023 blog post*[43]

During the darkest day of the pandemic, I started keeping a gratitude journal. I was inspired to do so by Janice Kaplan's enlightening book, *The Gratitude Diaries*, in which she chronicled her year-long journey focused on cultivating gratitude. Through insightful research and personal reflections, Kaplan's exploration of the transformative power of gratitude deeply affected my understanding of its significance and potential in our lives.

However, the nature of our work as doctors prevents us from maintaining a constant state of gratitude. The relentless exposure to suffering and death makes trite phrases like "Everything happens for a reason" seem woefully inadequate in providing comfort or understanding. Dr. Susan David's groundbreaking work on emotional agility has significantly influenced my perspective, encouraging me to advocate for its integration into medical education. In her acclaimed book *Emotional Agility*, Dr. David wisely dissects the pervasiveness of toxic positivity within American culture. She explores the persistent influence of social media and well-intentioned individuals who advocate simplistic mantras like "Smile" or "There's always something to be thankful for," highlighting the limitations and potential harm associated with such approaches.

Any great therapist will highlight the importance of acknowledging and processing our emotions. Regrettably, this critical understanding eluded me until well after my residency. It remains a significant deficiency in our medical education system. We must be adequately equipped with the tools to navigate and manage our emotional landscapes effectively. However, I hold no ill will toward my educators. As Maya Angelou once wisely proclaimed, "Do the best you can until you know better. Then, when you know better, do better." We know better now, and our medical professionals and our patients deserve to be treated by clinicians with emotional agility. We need and deserve doctors who can sit with us compassionately and shift into an analytical and thoughtful state. Then, perhaps ten minutes later, exchange lighthearted moments with a colleague, much like learning to ride a wave when surfing (or paddleboarding, in my case), it takes great skill to ride the big waves.

Medicine regularly immerses us in the most profound and intense moments of individuals' lives. Each day brings the responsibility of delivering life-altering news, the weight of which lingers long after the moment has passed. The memory of sitting with a grieving mother, delivering the devastating news of her child's death, remains engraved in my consciousness, a permanent reminder of the emotional toll of our profession.

The scope of education regarding processing difficult emotions typically revolved around a generalized acknowledgment of the challenges inherent in our roles as doctors. For a lot of our medical training, it was pretty much "get back on the horse" after a sad case or a bad outcome. There is little instruction on how to get back on. We are told to just get on it. Worse, if you struggle to get back on, we'll shame you for not being professional or strong. While a more supportive environment might encourage seeking assistance when needed, there is a notable absence of guidance based on insights from the psychological community on managing and processing these intense, emotional experiences effectively.

In line with Dr. David's research, the only viable pathway to navigate through and beyond the depths of an emotion is to confront it. No amount of toxic positivity or immersion in the mantra of "this is what doctors do" can shield us from the raw impact of these emotional encounters.

While it remains undeniable that it is a profound privilege to be present with individuals during their most vulnerable moments, I honestly cannot confess to feeling gratitude when tasked with delivering devastating news. Bad things happen, and sitting with someone and trying to make the worst day a little better is a privilege.

Dr. David advocates embracing emotional agility, emphasizing it is not about adopting an unfeeling, stoic demeanor. Instead, it entails allowing ourselves to experience and navigate our emotions. This, she suggests, is the fundamental key to effectively fulfilling the demands of this profession.

Amid the harrowing challenges brought forth by the pandemic, I realized the importance of acknowledging that the pandemic was an overwhelmingly distressing and terrible experience. I do not find comfort in expressing gratitude for it. I mourn the loss of many patients and boil with anger over the proliferation of misinformation and disinformation that worsened the public health crisis, exposing both myself and my patients to high risks and emotional trauma.

I have learned the power of embracing "and." I can simultaneously grieve the passing of a patient *and* express gratitude for the exceptional teamwork that enabled us to provide the best care. I can be enraged by the chronic understaffing in our emergency departments *and* appreciate the significant meaning and impact of my demanding yet deeply fulfilling job. I can acknowledge my exhaustion *and* feel thankful for the comfort of returning to a beautiful home that my hard-earned job has afforded me.

The human tendency towards negativity bias is deeply rooted in our evolutionary history. It served as an essential mechanism for our survival, enabling us to remember potential dangers, poisonous plants, or encounters with threatening animals. However, in our modern lives, this negativity bias can be more of a hindrance than a help. In medicine, especially in emergency medicine, this bias is actively cultivated and constantly compels us to consider the worst-case scenarios for our patients. A routine illness could be a sign of a life-threatening condition, leading us down a path of cautious consideration.

Without conscious effort, this persistent negativity bias can shadow various aspects of our lives outside medicine. It becomes essential to counterbalance this bias with a mindful practice of gratitude. I call this practice "grounded gratitude," a genuine appreciation of our blessings. Even during some of the darkest moments of my life, I acknowledge the sheer difficulty of those times while remaining grateful for the simple comforts that surrounded me. Whether it was the comfort of my bed, the satisfaction of a delicious meal, the warmth of my dogs' affection, or the constant support of my husband, Chris, these elements consistently served as strong anchors in my life.

During the rough months of the pandemic, as I diligently tracked my expressions of gratitude, I noticed these recurring themes, reinforcing the significance of these simple yet essential sources of comfort in my life. They gave me much-needed stability and a sense of security during times of uncertainty.

Substantial evidence highlights gratitude's profound impact on our well-being. However, as doctors, we can sometimes feel obliged to engage in certain practices simply because they are expected of us. Starting a gratitude journal only out of obligation or expressing gratitude for a toxic job will not yield the desired benefits. Do not gaslight yourself. If you're not ready to start a gratitude practice, that's alright. Don't forget you could write everything you're upset about and hold space for a few things going okay, which may be as simple as the fact that you're breathing or can write words on a page. Sometimes, that's all we've got; even letting that little amount of light in can help.

When the time feels right, explore ways to express gratitude that genuinely resonate with you. While it is possible to find moments of thankfulness in solitude, consider opportunities for authentic and public displays of gratitude. Gratitude is contagious. Taking a break to sincerely express appreciation to a nurse who went the extra mile with a struggling patient to contribute to their treatment plan can have a lasting impact. Alongside showing gratitude, embracing mindfulness in these moments nurtures a healing environment, letting us fully immerse ourselves in the present without rushing to the next task.

In medicine, one phrase can instantly induce trepidation in most of us: "Do you remember that patient?" Typically, it is followed by a recount of how a patient "bounced back," indicating a re-presentation and insinuating that a diagnosis was missed or an error was made. As emergency doctors, we find ourselves particularly vulnerable to a barrage of criticisms from various individuals within the medical community, faulting us for ordering too many tests or not enough, all without acknowledging the hindsight bias. In the rapid and demanding environment of the emergency department, it's nearly impossible to make every diagnosis, and sometimes, the best course of action is to admit the patient for further examination.

This prevailing culture of primarily receiving feedback when we falter presents an opportunity for the infusion of gratitude. A powerful example of this was demonstrated by a cardiologist with whom I used to work. He sent me HIPAA-compliant text messages detailing the cardiac catheterization results of our patients. The message included a photo of the occluded and now-opened coronary artery and a note expressing gratitude for my contribution to the patient's positive outcome.

In one particular case, the patient arrived experiencing no chest pain, a far cry from the typical presentation of a heart attack. While in the emergency department, an electrocardiogram (EKG) was conducted, revealing the ST elevations that justified a "code STEMI," indicating an urgent need for cardiac catheterization. Given the absence of symptoms that would have immediately called for an EKG, the diagnosis was delayed. After receiving a text from the cardiologist, a wave of anxiety washed over me, only to be replaced with surprise as I read the message: "Good catch, that was a difficult diagnosis, and he had 100% occlusion of his left anterior descending (LAD, also known as the widow maker) coronary. Thanks for taking care of him." Even though more than a year has passed, recounting that incident still brings tears to my eyes.

After reflecting on my emotional response, I recognize that this colleague's simple act of kindness, generosity, and commendation struck me profoundly. Such displays of gratitude are often strange to us, making them all the more moving. Creating opportunities to spread gratitude within our workplaces is essential. While many organizations have committees, processes, and dedicated staff focused on addressing errors, could we also invest in system solutions that support the culture of gratitude?

Implementing a gratitude program serves as a prime example of reinforcing a Safety II culture. The fundamental principle of Safety II rests on recognizing that most of our responses to errors are rooted in Safety I, emphasizing a retrospective analysis of what went wrong. Regrettably, there is a lack of dedicated personnel and resources to foster a Safety-II approach that focuses on comprehending what went right. Gratitude initiatives exemplify how we can actively reinforce positive aspects within workplaces and organizations. For further insights into Safety II, listen to my interview on the Heartline podcast with Dr. Shannon McNamara, who introduced me to this concept along with resilience engineering.

Last, I must comment on the phrase, "Thank you for your service." This phrase has been said to me countless times. Sometimes, it has been said so quickly that it sounds like "Gesundheit" after someone sneezes. What I wanted, especially when I first came home, was not appreciation, expressed through the words "Thank you," I yearned for gratitude, which, in the book *Atlas of the Heart*, Dr. Brené Brown describes gratitude as a practice, more than simply uttering thanks. We have a lot of performative appreciation in our society, including directed toward veterans. We also saw it directed to healthcare workers at the beginning of the pandemic. It's easy to put a yellow ribbon on your car. It's easy to bang pots together. Gratitude involves an action, and it may be small. It may be looking someone deeply in the eye. It may be pausing to receive a response, which, when I came home from deployment, was a mixture of sadness and exhaustion. Words matter a lot, even simple words like "Thank you." Taking a moment to look at people and acknowledge their presence when we say thank you or thanks is a start.

Expressing gratitude in real time may not always be feasible. However, the power of returning to someone to express gratitude, whether an hour, a day, a week or even much later, spanning several years, is not to be underestimated. Taking the time to pause and genuinely thank someone the following day, acknowledging their significant contributions to patient care or their role in your learning and growth, holds far greater value than leaving it unspoken.

Reflect:

1. Reflect on a time when you experienced genuine gratitude in your professional life. How did it feel? What were the circumstances surrounding it? How did it impact your well-being?

_____

_____

_____

2. Consider when you struggled to find gratitude amidst challenges or setbacks in your career. What barriers did you face in acknowledging and embracing gratitude in that

situation? How did it affect your overall well-being?

_____

_____

_____

Reimagine:

1. Imagine a scenario where you incorporate the practice of grounded gratitude into your daily routine. What does this look like for you? How does it influence your interactions with colleagues, patients, and yourself?

_____

_____

2. Envision a workplace culture where grounded gratitude is cultivated and celebrated. How does this environment promote well-being and healthy resilience? What strategies can be implemented to foster this culture?

_____

_____

_____

Respond:

Create a gratitude ritual or practice tailored to your life. Describe how you will implement this practice into your daily routine and the potential benefits you expect to experience from it.

_____

_____

_____

Resources:

Enhancing Fulfillment and Connection through Gratitude with Dr. Linda Lawrence. The Heartline podcast.

The Gratitude Diaries by Janice Kaplan.

Atlas of the Heart: Mapping Meaningful Connection and the Language of Human Experience by Brené Brown. p. 211-214

Getting Back to Homeostasis with Dr. Shannon McNamara. The Heartline podcast, Jun 28, 2022.

For further reading on Safety II, I recommend Ham DH. Safety-II and Resilience Engineering in a Nutshell: An Introductory Guide to Their Concepts and Methods. Saf Health Work. 2021;12(1):10-19.

CHAPTER 24

MUSIC AS THERAPY

"We let people pick music while getting ultrasound…we always had music playing in the OR…music is always there, and it's been a best friend to me." — Dr. Corinna Muller on Heartline podcast, Aug 8, 2023

Long commutes have become a welcomed refuge for processing the tough parts of being a doctor. There are evenings when I conclude my shift with a whirlwind of thoughts competing for my attention - questions about the accuracy of my diagnoses and concerns about the fate of the patients experiencing homelessness I've attended to dominate my mind. During these taxing moments, I discovered music's therapeutic power. Turning to my carefully curated favorite playlist, which has expanded to 475 songs, has become my go-to remedy. I've grown so intimately familiar with the lyrics and melodies of these songs I can recognize them within the first few beats, giving me a profound sense of comfort and grounding among the chaos.

One of the hardest parts of being a doctor is losing patients. For me, the patients that come in talking to me and later die leave a profound impact on me. To hear someone's voice, in addition to seeing their face, lays down more tracks of connection and memory, making their death more challenging than the patients that I never get to talk with due to the severity of their illness or injury.

I recall a patient in her 60s who came in with a heart attack. She cracked jokes with the team, and while her condition was serious, her joking put us all at ease. Some patients will also share facial expressions or characteristics that remind us of family members; here, she reminded me of my mom. Later in her stay, her heart stopped, and despite our best efforts, we couldn't get her back.

As I began the drive home that day, I thought about her voice. Then, my thoughts went to my mom, and I contemplated her age and mortality. I turned on my '70s playlist of songs I used to listen to my mom, and Crosby, Stills, and Nash's "We May Never Pass This Way Again" turned on. A few tears streamed down my face.

Anna Rainville (LMFT) shared that driving involves some of the same eye movements reported in eye movement desensitization and reprocessing therapy (EMDR). Driving and listening to therapeutic music can accelerate emotional processing. While more research is needed, there is a concept called mood-matching music to enhance emotional processing. In this school of thought, matching the music to your mood with the conscious thought of processing the related emotions can help alleviate difficult emotions. This differs from choosing a genre opposite to "cheer up," for example, choosing happy music if you're feeling sad.[44]

The key is probably what we've discussed in other sections of the book. If you put on a happy song, you may momentarily feel better, but the difficult emotion you're turning away from will probably still be there.

Music has become an integral part of my pre-shift routine, thanks to the insightful concept introduced by Dr. Joelle Bohart at the 2019 FeminEM Idea Exchange. Inspired by her idea of having a walk-up song, I carefully curated my playlist of refreshing tracks, each serving as a powerful tool for igniting my passion and enthusiasm. During moments when fatigue threatens to overshadow my anticipation for the upcoming shift, the empowering anthems of Destiny's Child, including the spirited "Independent Woman" and resilient "Survivor," along with the infectious energy of Lady Gaga's "Edge of Glory," serve as my motivational boost, fortifying me to embrace the challenges that lie ahead in the day (or night) to come. Before a night shift, I love listening to "Night Moves" by Bob Segar or "Takin' Care of Business" by Bachman-Turner Overdrive.

Following the pandemic, my first venture back into the world of live music was marked by an unforgettable evening with James Taylor. As the first chords of the performance echoed through the venue, a surge of emotion swept over me, provoking a waterfall of tears. The experience of reentering a bustling concert hall, accompanied by the familiar yet commanding presence of James Taylor's voice, stirred within me a profound sense of release and renewal, creating a liberating effect that resonated on multiple levels.

Since that transformative evening, I have actively pursued more opportunities to participate in live musical performances. Despite the considerable expense and occasional hurdles in navigating the commute to and from the venue, the collective ambiance of being surrounded by a crowd of individuals, all enraptured by the artist's spellbinding performance, is an immensely healing and revitalizing experience. An added joy of attending live concerts is the enduring ability to be transported back to those cherished moments whenever the familiar melodies grace my ears again.

Top 10 Soul Songs—narrowing it down to ten songs was hard. These are the songs that I can play on repeat when I'm feeling down and need to process something hard.

10. "Strong Enough," by Sheryl Crow

9. "Change is Gonna Come," by Leela James

8. "Remind Me," by Emily King

7. "Strength, Courage, and Wisdom," by India Arie

6. "Love is on the Way," by Billy Porter

5. "Hold On," by Wilson Phillips

4. "Right to be Wrong," by Joss Stone

3. "In Too Deep," by Genesis

2. "Drink Wine," by Adelle

1. "Closer to Fine," by the Indigo Girls

Top 10 Walk Up Songs:

10. "Girl on Fire," by Alicia Keys

9. "Don't Stop," by Fleetwood Mac

8. "Anticipation," by Carly Simon

7. "Good as Hell," by Lizzo

6. "I'm Every Woman," by Chaka Khan

5. "Can't Stop," by Red Hot Chili Peppers

4. "Up," by Shania Twain

3. "Start Me Up," by Rolling Stones

2. "Respect," by Aretha Franklin

1. "Don't You Worry 'Bout A Thing," by Stevie Wonder, is possibly my favorite song. I instantly start dancing anytime this song is on.

Reflect:

What are some of your favorite songs and artists? When do you turn to music in your life?

_____

_____

_____

Reimagine:

How could incorporating music more intentionally in healthcare impact the well-being of patients and healthcare workers?

_____

_____

_____

Respond:

Create your walk-up playlist for when you need to be pumped up for work. What other playlists would you like to create for your home or work to support emotional processing or for more enjoyment?

_____

_____

_____

Resources:

The Harmony of Healing with Dr. Corinna Muller, *Heartline* podcast. Episode 44.

You Need a Walk-Up Song by Joelle C. Bohart, MD. https://feminem.org/podcast/you-need-a-walk-up-song/

Andrea Austin

CHAPTER 25

HUMOR

"We all walk in with I'm a doctor…we lead with that…. improv lets me play this character, the one I choose to be in a way that is meaningful and authentic to me." — Dr. Wendy Schofer on Heartline podcast, Mar 12, 2024

My love for comedy is a heartfelt acknowledgment to my mom, who introduced me to its joys. Watching Seinfeld together holds some of my cherished childhood memories. The excitement of *Seinfeld* coming on prompted us to break into a funny dance, standing side by side, shaking our hips. Vague recollections exist of me cracking jokes as a kid. Those jokes probably garnered more laughter than expected because I likely infused them with the sarcasm and adult humor I absorbed (maybe a bit too early) from shows like *Frasier*, *Seinfeld*, and reruns of *The Mary Tyler Moore Show*. Lines delivered by a seven-year-old were probably amusing, or at least surprising!

However, I suppressed my inclination to tell jokes somewhere along the way. I started perceiving it as silly and rebellious, not aligning with the image of the "good girl" I aspired to be, both at home and in school. I let go of my fleeting dream of becoming a comedian and pivoted toward what I perceived as serious intellectual pursuits. In hindsight,

I could have been a good comedian. Comedians are clever, and I love wordplay. Interviewing Dr. Wendy Schofer, who shared her journey to lean into improv and stand-up, reminds me that maybe my time as a comedian hasn't fully passed me by yet.

Reflecting on medicine's hidden curriculum, which encompasses stoicism, perfectionism, and competition, it becomes clear that stoicism poses a significant challenge to infusing humor into the medical field. Despite this, humor remains an integral part of the human experience and has a natural way of surfacing.

One of my most cherished mentors, Dr. Gerald Platt, has a remarkable talent for injecting humor into medicine. I use the term "infusing" deliberately, as it's not akin to the humor-filled episodes of a show like *Scrubs*. Instead, he adeptly finds subtle ways to introduce lightheartedness. Thinking about the rules of comedy, either purposefully or accidentally, he follows many:

1. Don't punch down. Our patients come to us vulnerable, and while many of their problems could be funny (let's face it, an object in the rectum has an inherent bit of hee-hee-ness to it), it's not amusing to the person there in the bed, having to explain what is there and then deal with the consequences, which, under the worse

circumstances, may involve surgery.

2. It's okay to laugh *with*, not *at* people. It's similar to the don't punch down, but slightly different in that sometimes patients crack jokes (outstanding ones). Humor can be an adaptive coping mechanism, and bonding over the absurdity of a situation, a play on words, or embracing the silliness of our bodies can be fun. Somewhere along the way, due to an overemphasis on stoicism, I lost the ability to laugh with my patients. Part of the revitalization process has been embracing these moments of humor with my patients.

3. Be careful with sarcasm. Dr. Platt told me this early on, and I resisted as a devoted fan of *Seinfeld* and sarcasm. There are so many opportunities for sarcasm in medicine. If you'd like a master class, watch the attending physician, Perry Cox, on Scrubs. He exudes sarcasm with nearly every word he utters on the show, and I freaking love it.

While *Scrubs* offers an entertaining portrayal, it's essential to acknowledge that it diverges from real-life scenarios. Admitting this truth, after years of adopting a somewhat sarcastic approach as a doctor, I've agreed with Dr. Platt (for the most part). The issue with sarcasm lies in the underlying cynicism it carries. I liken sarcasm to a decadent dessert, which you know might lead to diabetes, covered in whipped cream and a thick layer of icing. Consume this dessert sparingly, just as you should use sarcasm about medicine infrequently.

Sarcasm often directs its punches downward, violating the first rule of comedy—don't punch down. So, how can one satisfy their appetite for smart comedy? Being clever and witty scratches the same itch without the inherent nastiness frequently embedded in sarcasm.

In the age of memes, a LOT of sarcasm is shared about medicine. In 2022, as I began the most challenging work of the revitalization period, I thought a lot about my social media consumption. One thing I noticed was that watching a lot of sarcastic videos and memes about medicine was adding to my apathy and "Everything is bullshit" attitude.

Please keep sending me your sarcastic memes, but know that I won't always like or laugh at them. I may ignore them for days or weeks, depending on my current mood and what I need. If I'm already teetering on, "Everything is bullshit, and I made the wrong choice going into medicine," then watching a sarcastic video feels good at the moment. Still, it isn't doing me any favors, as I try to get a good mood pre-shift or gear up for a long, and maybe not so gratifying meeting.

4. Timing is everything. We do hard, serious, and

often sad work. Dr. Platt is SO funny; he also has high emotional intelligence. He knows when to use humor and when to be serious. He is also among the most thoughtful and intensely serious-when-necessary people I know. Read the room and understand that what you think is funny, or when you might be open to a joke, may differ from everyone else. This is important when working with medical trainees. Often, what may seem minor or an opportunity for humor, for them, seems high stakes and is anything but funny. Go back to rules 1 and 2: don't punch down and laugh with and not at anyone.

5. Props (or the lack of props) can be hilarious. As discussed earlier in the book, simulations are vital for training medical students and residents. Dr. Platt directed a lot of the simulations when I was a resident. When we'd get to the part of the scenario where we'd need to call a consultant, the resident would say, "I want to talk to cardiology." He'd say, "Well, I can't get the cardiologist until you pick up the phone." The resident would say, "What phone?" Then, Dr. Platt would hold his small finger next to his mouth and thumb next to his ear, the universal (at least in the US) sign for a phone, and then, the resident would do the same thing. It was silly. In a humorous way, it acknowledged that we were in a simulated

environment.

Humor as a key element to doctoring is not just a laughing matter (yes, I realize that's a stupid pun, but as a lover of puns, even bad ones like that, it's staying in the book, despite the multiple suggested cuts by my editor). There is a growing appreciation that improv has a role in educating doctors. To be a good improv actor, you must listen to your other actors and react, the golden rule being the "Yes and" approach to an excellent improv skit. As doctors, we improv all the time. I can't tell you how many times I've walked into a room; the chief complaint on the chart says one thing, and the patient says something different. I had to scrap the script and improv my way through the visit. As with comedy, the improvisation becomes easier with lots of practice. While I may not have seen this exact combination of complaints, I have enough experience to get through the visit, and if I'm really on my game, get the patient to relax, smile, and maybe even laugh.

Let's talk about gallows humor. It's a real thing. I was a medical student the first time I heard someone make a sick joke (sick in the awful, gross, not cool sick way). I remember thinking how rude and unprofessional it was and that patients would hate us if they heard it. Then, and sadly, not after too long, I would join in. Sadly, medicine has elements of gang culture. You learn to get along; you've got to go along. The medical student is so far down the pecking order, way below the nurse, and for the *Scrubs* fan, the janitor gets more respect, so anything you can do to get in with the cool residents or attendings, you do. Gallows humor is an example of humor that punches down.

When you listen to gallows humor and watch it done, it's clear, after years of therapy, that it is a maladaptive coping mechanism. Thus, instead of scolding everyone for their unprofessional behavior, gallows humor is an opportunity to check in on a colleague. Do you know what cuts gallows humor with a knife? Vulnerability. When someone makes a joke about how if the patient were serious about killing themselves, they would have done it the right way (yes, this is a realistic, horrifically cringy comment that happens), it's an opportunity to say an authentic, vulnerable response. For example, any patient with a suicide attempt, even those that are considered "gestures," a horrible term used for when a suicide attempt is considered not significant enough to result in a life-threatening illness or injury, is more likely to die from suicide.

Reflecting on what made COVID-19 so shitty (there are not enough pages for that book), one of them for us doctors was it was hard to laugh. Laughter is contagious, and having our mouths covered by masks made it hard to connect and laugh. I don't know if I ever laughed while I had my N-95 on. Maybe a funny patient or colleague would transmit enough of their laugh lines and eye twinkle under the rarest circumstances to get a stifled chuckle.

Plenty has been written on laughter as medicine. Laughter is associated with reduced cortisol, the hormone related to stress.[45] Some of my favorite moments have involved laughing to the point of feeling like I can't breathe, a particular form of laugh-hyperventilation, or spitting out a beverage.

Reflect: Recall a time when humor helped you navigate a stressful or challenging situation. How did it change your perspective or alleviate your stress? What kind of humor was most effective for you?

_____

_____

_____

Reimagine: Envision incorporating more laughter into your days. How could you use humor to diffuse tension and foster a more positive work and home environment? What specific strategies or practices can you adopt?

_____

_____

_____

Respond: Identify three ways you can bring more joy into your life this week. Whether it's through watching a funny show, sharing jokes with colleagues, or finding humor in everyday situations, write down your plan and how you will implement it.

_____

_____

_____

Resources:

Accepting Burnout to Find Your Path: A Pediatrician Learns Integrity and Revitalization Through Play with Dr. Wendy Schofer. *Heartline* podcast. Episode 67.

Kramer CK, Leitao CB. Laughter as medicine: A systematic review and meta-analysis of interventional studies evaluating the impact of spontaneous laughter on cortisol levels. *PLoS One.* 2023;18(5): e0286260. Published 2023 May 23. doi:10.1371/journal.pone.0286260

Andrea Austin

CHAPTER 26

THE REVITALIZED HEALER

"When people are hurt, they need someone that is caring and warm. You don't need to be a blanket, but you can extend one."
— Dr. Katrina Landa on Heartline podcast May 31, 2022

I want to return to compassion in medicine and the idea that to survive in medicine, we must become hardened, and thus, our compassion will dissipate. I no longer feel that losing our compassion is inevitable; to be fulfilled and serve our patients, our compassion is not a nice thing to have; it's essential.

From my own experience, compassion diminishes from two primary causes. First, there is the idea of compassion fatigue, which gained much recognition during the pandemic. When we continue to pour from an empty cup, exhaustion can extinguish the flame of compassion. We need time to connect with our patients to form empathic bonds and to recover from difficult moments. Our compassion erodes without the time to connect with our patients and reconnect with ourselves.

I have also felt my compassion decrease as a preemptive, protective strategy. I have "armored up" before going into a tough situation, distancing myself from the patient and reducing my compassion. The armor also prevents us from feeling the support of colleagues. Thus, compassion requires Olympic-level emotional agility. As Dr. Omar Reda reminds us, we must prepare to be wounded. Yet, these wounds are not all ugly or necessarily bad. They help us form connections. When we recognize them and seek support and time to recover, we can be even more effective caregivers.

To understand compassion, we must explore a key ingredient: empathy. Empathy is the capacity to comprehend and share the feelings of others. Considering our work in medicine, trying to envision the emotional and physical agony associated with illnesses such as cancer can be distressing. I use the term "painful" not as a metaphor but rather as a reflection of the fact that functional MRI data shows that when we try to imagine the suffering of others, it activates the pain pathway in our brains.[46]

After almost a decade of practicing medicine as an empath, I felt like a dishtowel that had been squeezed too many times. I realized that I couldn't continue my job in the same way that had led me to this point.

As this realization unfolded, Sharee Johnson, psychologist and coach, introduced me to the concept that rather than simply being empathic, it's more effective to approach our role as caregivers with compassion.

Compassion embodies empathy along with an active response. This action could be as simple as listening to a patient or as significant as performing a life-saving procedure like placing a tube to relieve pressure in the chest. The important part is recognizing the compassionate action grounded in empathy. Compassion triggers the reward centers of our brain, leading to the release of dopamine, our brain's "feel-good" chemical.

Likely well-meaning, we downplay the importance of a healthy ego to avoid selfishness and narcissism. Many doctors I know will minimize the awesomeness of what they do, asserting that "it's what anyone with our training would do." Yet, medicine still requires skill and courage. Failing to acknowledge our contributions drives a loss of personal efficacy. Finding the balance between humility and a healthy sense of pride is vital in addressing the apathy and reduced sense of achievement associated with burnout. In Alison Levine's book, *On the Edge*, she discusses how Coach Krzyzewski from the Duke men's basketball team wants players with a healthy ego. This balance of ego is succinctly described in Dr. Brené Brown's *The Gifts of Imperfection* as the phrase, "Don't shrink. Don't puff up. Stand your sacred ground." Learning to hold both while healing: to be humble yet exerting a healthy amount of pride about what you do is integral to thriving.

Part of the reason that many doctors struggle with this

balance of ego is that we don't explicitly talk about it in medical training. All too often, we don't have great role modeling. Many doctors will emulate the "puff up" style by yelling, demeaning, and other acts to exert their ego. At the same time, others are meek and let people step all over them. Dr. Brown's phrase, "…stand your sacred ground," is profound when applying it to healthcare. There is no need to puff up if you're standing your ground, squarely on the sacredness of healing and advocating for your patients. The nobility of that action speaks for itself, regardless of whether the receiver believes that or provides validation.

When you believe, in your heart and mind, that you're following your heartline and no longer rely on your self-worth being connected to others, you can be an inspired and profoundly resilient healer. You'll be able to have a strong back, soft heart (a common phrase in meditation), and follow your heartline. When more of us start doing this, healthcare will have to change. The system is made of people, and we can change it. Change starts within us and impacts teams, and these ripples become waves that transform the broader organization.

***

Somewhere along the way, many healers forget the profound impact of the therapeutic relationship. The simple act of listening can be immensely healing. In addition to the fight-or-flight response, the tend-and-befriend response is also a coping mechanism. Tending and befriending, with boundaries, can be a highly adaptive way to cope with the stresses of caregiving. Genuine human connection leads to the release of oxytocin, a hormone associated with well-being and bonding. Recognizing the dual nature of the therapeutic relationship has been crucial in my doctoring journey. During the darkest days of the COVID-19 pandemic, it felt like patients were an outsized source of physical or emotional harm. Now, I appreciate that in addition to healing them, these interactions have the potential to enhance my well-being and personal growth.

As I revised this book, a recent patient impacted me. He was in his early twenties and presented with new-onset diabetes, which was making him critically ill. We worked to get IVs on him for many minutes, and it was clear that he was too dehydrated for us to access the usual vessels and that we'd have to perform an invasive procedure called a central line. As the resident prepared to place the line, I went to the head of the bed and calmly spoke to the patient, reassuring him we would get him through this illness. I may have been more detached in earlier years, but this time, I leaned into the hard part; caring for this patient was easier, not harder.

Yet, while I rode this emotional wave, our teamwork made navigating it easier. We had several minutes to huddle after the case to debrief. We offered words of encouragement and gratitude to each other. In contrast to some nights, where I am the only physician present, it's hard to process emotions while simultaneously leaving enough cognitive capacity to do the work. Safely containing and flagging these emotions tied to these situations to process later, rather than unconsciously detaching, is the best approach. I'll unpack safely containing more through an example.

Picture yourself examining a three-year-old child with multiple burns. According to the mother, these burns resulted from a curling iron falling off the vanity. However, the burn locations don't align with the provided story. As a mandatory reporter, you are responsible for reporting potential abuse. Unfortunately, social work is unavailable, and you alone must inform the mother that a mandatory report will be filed with child protective services, prompting her to lash out at you. She questions your intentions and clinical judgment. The confrontation leaves you feeling anxious and emotionally wounded.

As you exit the room, a nurse alerts you that a patient in room 10 is experiencing respiratory distress. The resuscitation effort culminates in the patient being intubated, along with emotionally charged conversations with the patient's family. This chaotic scenario unfolds right before shift change, and your replacement scrutinizes your plans for several other patients. You experience a feeling of shame for not being adequately prepared for the turnover, rather than self-compassion, recognizing no one could have been more prepared given what unfolded so close to shift change. You take getting a verbal dressing down by a colleague in front of the team and don't push back in the moment or take him off to the side later to discuss how this interaction impacted you. Resentment and frustration build.

Exhausted and disheartened, you make your way to your car, the details of the night blurring due to your fatigue. You briefly contemplate confiding in your friend Ann, who has always been understanding, but it's already 10 p.m. Upon reaching home, you grab some chips and turn on Netflix. Two hours later, you awaken on the couch and walk up to your bed.

The following day, over coffee with your partner, he asks about your shift. You reply, "It was hectic, more of the usual." You head out for a run, your mind drifting to thoughts of your upcoming vacation. That evening, as you step in for another shift, the nurse informs you about an upset mother at the triage desk, threatening to leave with her child, having waited only 15 minutes. With five new patients to attend to in your designated area, one exhibiting a troubling EKG, you feel anger as you rush to the front. While you understand the frustration of waiting in the emergency department with a sick child, you can't help feeling annoyed by the mother's lack of situational awareness, considering the nature of an emergency room.

What just happened? Being well-rested and recovered and having addressed the challenging emotions from the previous shift would enable one to display the best self, approach the frustrated mother with compassion, and likely de-escalate the situation swiftly. However, in this case, the mother's frustration and rudeness are not only tied to this interaction. Instead, this interaction triggers the unresolved feelings associated with the mother from last night's incident.

So, what's the solution? In emergency medicine and many other professions, we lack the luxury of instantly processing every emotion we experience. Often, for the safety of our patients and those around us, we must compartmentalize our feelings. During training, this was frequently described as "pushing through it." We also use terms like "grinding it out." Although not an ideal practice, it is the reality of what is required of us. Psychologists suggest that a more adaptive approach is safely containing rather than compartmentalization.

When dealing with trauma, it is widely recognized that discussing traumatic events can trigger heightened emotional distress and symptoms of posttraumatic stress. In the context of EMDR, one of the initial techniques taught involves placing distressing memories related to trauma into a designated safe container. The safe container is created visually during an early session, often represented by an imagined secure location within one's home where valuable possessions or documents would be kept, such as an actual safe.

How can we implement this technique practically? Let's consider the mother yelling at me about the mandatory report. As I exit the room and transition into caring for the critical patient, I mentally envision placing that recent interaction into my safe container, which is a safe located in my home.

How does this method differ from my previous approach following challenging encounters? When something is stored in a safe, it remains accessible and retrievable. It is not repressed, suppressed, or numbed. It is set aside for later reflection when I have the time, privacy, and mental and physical energy to process the event.

What should you place in your safe? Well, it differs for each individual. Recall Faith Harper's definition of trauma from her book *UnF*ck Your Brain*: trauma is anything that significantly affects you. You have the right to define what qualifies as significant. It's essential to recognize that even something seemingly minor can impact you profoundly, depending on factors such as your sleep, past traumas, and emotional capacity for the day. Avoid comparing your traumas to determine if they merit a place in the safe. For example, saying, "I shouldn't be so disturbed by that interaction. I should be grateful for my job; it's not like my life was in danger or I'm in a war zone." This comparison game is a defense mechanism and delays healing.

How should you handle what's in your safe? This question is best answered by you, possibly with the guidance of a therapist. Simply taking them out and reflecting on them the following day might be enough for minor traumas. Consider journaling or confiding in a trusted friend or colleague to talk it through. However, if an event triggers memories of past traumas, such as the yelling mother bringing up childhood experiences, seeking assistance from a therapist may be necessary to work through these complex emotions.

Lastly, bottom-up strategies for processing trauma involving movement, such as yoga, dance, or even literally shaking it out for a moment, are also invaluable. If you think shaking it out sounds weird, watch some nature videos of animals that escape the snarls of predators. Once in a safe location, they may have uncontrollable shaking, which is reported as a way of "shaking off" the trauma. Thus, even at work, you could walk outside and gaze at the horizon, an example of a centering practice, followed by shaking your body for a few seconds. The practices are maneuvers to let some steam out of our proverbial pot about to boil over. In

Burnout: The Secret to Unlocking the Stress Cycle, the Nagoski sisters discuss this in more detail and emphasize that movement is the most efficient way to complete a stress cycle, aka process something.

On an intellectual level, we may understand that hurtful comments or actions by patients or colleagues are not about us. Yet, that doesn't prevent the emotional impact on us. No amount of rationalization can eliminate the inherent emotional aspect of our work, which intersects with the narrative of our own lives. If you've been relying on rationalization to navigate these experiences, I urge you to consider this strategy's effectiveness. For many of us, using rationalization is a defense mechanism that hinders us from confronting the necessary task of processing our challenging emotions. So, the next time you tumble down the rabbit hole of rationalization, take a moment to pause and contemplate whether it might be more appropriate to place it in the safe and commit to carving out time to process it.

Physicians are skilled at compartmentalizing. We can seamlessly transition from delivering devastating news to a family to engaging in playful interactions with a child—the necessity of managing these interactions swiftly and with emotional flexibility demands that we compartmentalize. However, we must not deceive ourselves; every act of compartmentalization leaves an imprint. It's akin to emptying the contents of a vacuum cleaner into the trash. A small puff of dust always surfaces. Invisible, this dust or residue can transfer to the next person. Over time, these nearly invisible particles accumulate, forming layers that affect us. We must shift from compartmentalizing to safely containing and processing our experiences.

The medical hierarchy exalts expertise while disregarding the novice. Through my engagement with the Recalibrate© program,[47] I understand that cultivating a beginner's mindset is essential for maintaining longevity as a doctor. One effective way I access the beginner's mind is by surrounding myself with individuals new to the field. Their fresh perspective helps me recapture the excitement of encountering a patient with chest pain for the first time. Observing the spark in their eyes and hearing the enthusiasm in their voices gives me a small dose of the wonder that what we do is remarkable.

While I was in the military, I learned the expression, "The beatings will stop when morale improves." We get programmed to think that the way to improve is by criticizing ourselves and others. Instead, we must cultivate self-compassion as the precursor to compassion for others.

If this is surprising or you're struggling with where to start, imagine how you would respond to a small child or a loved one if they made a mistake. Generally, we can be more compassionate to others than ourselves, and stepping out (a term from Dr. Susan David) and imagining how we'd react to someone else gets us on the fast track to self-compassion.

If I have one regret from both my deployment and the pandemic, it is I did not understand the Buddhist principle introduced to me by The Whole Physicians and the Recalibrate© program:

Pain = Resistance x Suffering

Suffering is inevitable. It is a part of the human experience. I'm reminded by Dr. Susan David's explanation that to expect that we won't feel angry, sad, or discomfort in life equals "dead people goals." The expectation to not suffer is not compatible with life. As Dr. Susan David explains, bottling or stuffing emotions will not make them disappear. Instead, they compound. We need to radically accept the emotion as information (not a directive to follow), refrain from judgment about having the emotion, experience it, and choose how we want to respond to act following our values. I can't tell you that moving through emotions is always fun. Many are painful and hard work. Yet, when we bottle or stuff emotions, we are delaying the inevitable. They also have a way of escaping in destructive and uncomfortable ways that can wreak havoc in our lives.

Resistance is alluring, though. As someone who gravitates more toward anger, resistance feels active. By resisting the emotion, I feel like I'm telling the person, the universe, that I am a fighter. Temporarily, this fighting energy feels good.

It is important to emphasize that allowing suffering and inviting negative emotions is separate from accountability. There is still much room for accountability. Seek justice and work for change. When you process your feelings, your changemaking ability strengthens.

Dr. Brené Brown closed one of her podcasts,[48] with a beautiful gift that changed my life. She shared the concept of how to live BIG, which stands for boundaries, integrity, and gratitude. In the episode, she explored the question, "Are people doing the best they can in life?" Dr. Brown's research showed that most people, after careful introspection, will conclude that people are doing the best that they can. Looking back on moments in my life in which I let myself or someone else down, I can conclude that I had an unmet need that contributed to me falling short. The question to continually return to, especially if you are in service to others, is, what do I need to show up to every day to stay within my boundaries, integrity, and gratitude?

How does this look for healers? The road to living BIG is paved through embodiment. Connect with your body. How do you feel? Return to the mnemonic introduced earlier in the book: PHAALLTS. I invite you to consider the times you haven't been compassionate to others. If you reflect on those moments, I suspect you will uncover that you didn't have what you needed to be compassionate. Maybe you were late, including being time-pressured, a common problem in healthcare and our fast-paced world.

Sometimes, I come home and tell my husband a harrowing story about my day. I sometimes tear up or share a soul-level feeling of exhaustion. He replies, "What you do is meaningful. And that's not a small thing."

He's articulating back what Dr. Susan David says: this is the price of admission. There is a path in which we can practice medicine BIG, within our boundaries, with integrity and gratitude. I will spend the rest of my career finding more ways to empower healers to live BIG earlier in their careers and help drive the changes in the system to support the well-being of our healthcare workers, not as a luxury but as the clear path to taking great care of patients.

Putting it all together:

Case 1: A 41-year-old woman presents to the emergency department with the worst headache of her life. Due to overcrowding, she was on a gurney in the hallway when I first examined her. Her vital signs are notable for high blood pressure, otherwise unremarkable. She's holding her head, and there's anguish across her face and in her voice as she describes the debilitating headache. As I listened to her, my heart beat faster, and it felt heavy. There is a sinking feeling in my stomach. While her neurological exam is normal, I sense there is a bleed in her brain. The emergency department was busy, so I quickly called radiology to expedite her scan and make the diagnosis. There is resistance to moving her to the front of the line, but I stand firm in advocating for my patient while staying calm and professional.

The nurse returns and tells me there is a large bleed. She asks, "How did you know? Her neurological exam is normal."

"I had a feeling; it was a mix of her story, tone, and vital signs that concerned me."

Reflecting later, I recall being embodied during the initial conversation with the patient. I didn't resist the pain I felt when hearing her story. I channeled it to do compassionate acts, expedite her CT scan, and order pain and blood pressure medicine.

Case 2: A 55-year-old male with a history of coronary artery bypass graft five years ago presents with right leg pain. He points to the scar on his right leg and spends several minutes recounting his harrowing experience with open heart surgery and his concerns that his leg pain is a sign that something is wrong with his heart. He is so anxious that I can feel my body vibrating in a similar heightened state. I'm mindful of what I'm feeling and reflect back to the patient that I'm sensing his anxiety. I also acknowledge his pain and understandable concern for a severe health problem. His speech begins to slow down. Together, we formulate a plan to check for the most serious causes of his leg pain.

When I return to share his normal results, I sense an opening to talk more directly about his anxiety and potential unprocessed emotional trauma due to his near-death experience. As I speak more slowly, his speech slows. As I talk softer, he talks softer. This is not magic but rather a very predictable response from neuroscience literature. We have mirror neurons programmed to respond similarly to those around us.

Furthermore, drawing on Polyvagal theory, I recognize that our nervous systems are programmed to co-regulate. This theory, developed by Dr. Stephen Porges[49], explains how our nervous system can get hijacked by trauma. While neuroscience has not substantiated Polyvagal theory on an anatomical level, it still provides a helpful conceptual framework for understanding psychological and physiological responses. Our autonomic nervous system (ANS) connects our brains and bodies. Think about how quickly your body can sense if you've touched something hot. This rapidity is lifesaving. Yet, the speed in our nervous system responses can be harmful when linked to triggers that no longer threaten us or to things that remind us of those triggers.

The framework Polyvagal theory provides allowed me to stay compassionate in the moment. I recognized that the patient was in a fight-or-flight state, evident by his anxiousness. The other portions of the polyvagal continuum include the dorsal vagal component, which, similar to fight-or-flight, is associated with self-protection. Rather than running or fighting, the dorsal vagal is in shutdown mode and shows up as numbing or other behaviors involving isolation.

Thankfully, I recalled that we are hard-wired for connection and healing, thanks to the ventral vagal nervous system response. This system is engaged through grounding practices, such as expressing gratitude and mindfulness, and acts of connection, such as smiling and hugging, all of which release oxytocin.

I shared that I've had a few traumas in my life as well and that therapy has been helpful. I wrote down the names of some books that helped me heal. There was a palpable sense of calm and connection in the room.

A few minutes later, I saw the patient walking out of the emergency department holding the hand of his granddaughter. She stopped, turned, and said, "Thank you, doctor." I tear up for a minute because while they thought this was a unidirectional moment of healing, in fact, it was healing to me as well.

As I returned to my desk, I paused and reflected. I recall an article shared by the Physician Coaching Institute on physician identity. For most of our medical training, we are encouraged to be fixers. Yet, much of what we encounter cannot be fixed. We can always heal. Many within the medical establishment look down on the word healing. It sounds soft and not evidence-based. I chose to use the word healing in the byline of this book, and I'm taking the time to unpack it here because setting down the identity of fixer and embracing healer is a much more sustainable path. It allows for the potential for patients to have much knowledge of their bodies and for us to partner together to strive for healing. Their desires around healing may be very different than what I think would "fix" them. With these realizations, I recognize that my brain is changing. I continue to learn and accumulate more experiences, and my mind and, most importantly, my heart expands. This revitalization helps me to keep doing the healing work for myself and my patients.

These case studies show how combining the critical concepts in this book—embodiment, compassion, and agency—is integral to revitalizing medicine. Leaning into the emotional part of healing requires the emotional intelligence and connectedness that patients and healthcare professionals crave on a soul level.

Returning to the question I'm frequently asked today: how long does it take to recover from burnout? That is only a question that you can answer yourself. Return to this book often. There are many different paths to following your heartline, and your reflections on the various prompts will continue to evolve over your life.

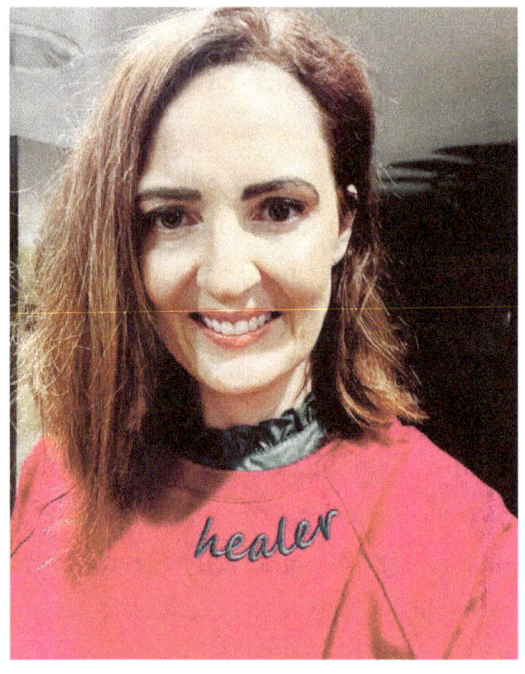

Revitalized Healer: scrubs and sweatshirt by GreenCloud apparel.

Reflect:

How do empathy and compassion manifest in your medical practice? Is there room to cultivate more compassion to enhance the fulfillment you experience as a healer?

_____

_____

_____

Reframe:

Think of a situation that is draining you while doctoring. It could be a particular type of patient you must interact with or task. Is there any way to reframe it into a compassionate act to make it more meaningful? For example, it is draining to see patients who ask for opioid prescriptions. The opioid epidemic has been devastating, and the opioids are so addictive. While I can hold the boundary around not prescribing opioids inappropriately, I can also do a compassionate act of connecting this patient with resources to help with their addiction.

_____

_____

_____

Reimagine:

Is there a way that you can help other healers in your work environment to understand empathy vs compassion and how to put this into practice?

_____

_____

_____

Resources:

On the Edge: Leadership Lessons from Mount Everest and Other Extreme Environments by Alison Levine.

Burnout: The Secret to Unlocking the Stress Cycle by Emily Nagoski and Amelia Nagoski.

The Thriving Doctor: How to be more balanced and fulfilled, working in medicine by Sharee Johnson.

Sharee Johnson: How Physicians Can Regain Agency & Lead. *Heartline* podcast. Episode 17.

Helping, Fixing, or Serving? Rachel Naomi Remen, Shambhala Sun, September 1999, was introduced to me by the Physician Coaching Institute.

EPILOGUE

WHERE DO WE GO FROM HERE?

Wellness 1.0 placed the onus of well-being solely on the healthcare professional, suggesting that individual actions like practicing yoga were enough to foster well-being– this was inherently flawed. Wellness 2.0 recognizes the resilience of healthcare workers and advocates for a renewed focus on system-level solutions to improve the well-being of workers and patients alike.

In its current form, the healthcare system is unsafe for both patients and healthcare workers. Yet, we need healthcare workers to continue to go to work every day, knowing they will face a range of occupational hazards, from workplace violence to circadian sleep disturbance linked to many health problems and exposure to infectious diseases, to name a few.

We have a significant task to reimagine and reshape healthcare for patients and workers. We must recognize that healthcare professionals are whole people with lives beyond their workplaces; they aren't superheroes. They need rest and support to navigate the challenges of being in their field. They need free and confidential mental healthcare to process the inherent trauma of their roles. In addition, coaching is a powerful way to support healthcare worker growth and contribute to the revitalization of healthcare.

How do we fund healthcare workers' access to mental health care? My veteran experience provides a tangible solution. The Vet Center is a community-based mental health network supported by an act of Congress recognizing the impact of the Vietnam War on veterans and their high rates of PTSD. We are in a similar moment; the healthcare workforce was strained pre-COVID, and COVID-19 has contributed significantly to a crisis in mental health among healthcare workers. Using the Vet Center model as a template, healthcare organizations could fund a network of mental healthcare practices specializing in healthcare workers' care. These funds would go to a system that operates independently from healthcare organizations to ensure free, confidential care for healthcare workers.

It is also time for accrediting bodies, such as The Joint Commission on Accreditation of Healthcare Organizations (JCAHO), to require public reporting and accountability for healthcare workers' well-being. When JCAHO or similar bodies visit a healthcare organization, and there is a violation or deviation from set standards, they require the healthcare organization to provide an action plan. They also follow up to ensure compliance. Specifically, the Well-Being Index by Mayo Clinic is a validated tool of healthcare professional well-being that can guide organizations towards actualizing a thriving workforce. It is also necessary that this information is publicly reported so that prospective employees can review it and consider it in their employment choices. In addition, like a Google review, patients should be able to see well-being rankings and make informed choices about where they get their healthcare. We need a race to the top, with organizations competing to be the best places for patient care and healthcare workers' well-being.

In addition, expanding the role of medical simulation is one powerful way to improve our organizations' safety, quality, and culture. We wouldn't get on a plane with pilots unless they had regular simulator refresher training. Why do we tolerate healthcare that doesn't leverage the power of simulation to acquire and maintain the knowledge, skills, and attitudes necessary for safe and quality care?

As I finished this book, I spoke with my dear friend, Jen (RA from chapter 3). We both studied biology and pre-med. Jen chose a different career path and later became a mother as well. There had always been a part of me that wondered if I should have pivoted away from pre-med, too, especially when thinking about how hard different aspects of being a doctor had been. As we said goodbye, I heard her daughter in the background and remarked, "Jen, I think you picked the better path than me." She usually laughs off such comments, but this time, she insisted it was not a better path, just different. Reflecting on my childhood dream of becoming a writer and despite winning a young writer's award, the dream withered, partly because I listened to those who discouraged me from being a writer and let medicine consume me. At that moment, looking out at my backyard and talking with my friend Jen, I realized that I had become a writer after all, and this more wholehearted way of living didn't take away from doctoring; instead, it made doctoring more fulfilling! I am revitalized.

Follow your heartline,

Andrea Austin, MD

ACKNOWLEDGMENTS

There are not enough pages to list the countless friends, mentors, and colleagues who have supported me. I want to mention a few that have been particularly impactful:

This book would not have happened without the wisdom and coaching of Sharee Johnson. She opened my eyes to how I could reconnect with the doctor I want to be and redesign my career to honor the doctor I am becoming.

Jen Hardy for her amazing friendship. I'm not always the easiest person, and Jen has shown me amazing grace and love throughout the years.

Dr. June Yoshii is a dear friend and colleague. Ten years after graduating from medical school, we lived in the same city and supposedly had our "dream jobs." Yet, we confided that there had to be something more. This conversation, compounded by years of others, was part of the push that helped me go from surviving to thriving.

Dr. Emi Latham. It's rare and special when you make friends with an attending physician. Thanks for being my teacher, and now my friend, travel companion, and supporter.

Lindsey Trout Hughes for her revising and editing services. She has a beautiful spirit, and her words of encouragement along this process were invaluable.

I am forever grateful to my incredible network of women veterans.

While the names are too numerous, there are a few that have had an outsized impact through friendship and mentorship: Dr. Danielle Wickman, Dr. Lisa Zaleski-Larsen, Dr. Loretta Stein, Dr. Torree McGowan, Dr. Katrina Landa, Dr. Amy Hildreth, Dr. Ann Long, Dr. Katie Ross, and Dr. Meaghan Kelville. We have shared laughs and tears, and we are forever trauma-bonded. I wouldn't choose the traumas again, but I'm forever thankful that it led to us becoming soul sisters.

Dr. Kerry King, Dr. Gerald Platt, Dr. Chris Chisholm, Dr. Michael Matteucci, Dr. Shaun Carstairs, Dr. Josh Hartzell and Dr. John Love for your mentorship, sponsorship and allyship. While there is still a long way to go in the military as whole for providing a safe and supportive environment for women, all of you are walking the walk.

Anna Rainville is a licensed Marriage and Family Therapist (LMFT) and Co-Owner and Clinical Director of Grounded Roots Mental Health Therapy. She is my friend and listened wholeheartedly to me early in my healing journey. She opened my eyes (pun intended) to EMDR and provided a necessary push to try it out.

Carmel Moreno is my friend and hairstylist. It is never just about hair; it is about healing and connection.

I'm thankful to the Vet Center, a phenomenal organization providing veterans with free mental healthcare. The two therapists I've worked with there have genuinely changed my life, and the insights shared in this book were informed through these sessions. My experience with the Vet Center has been remarkable. Each time I've shown up, I've been greeted with kindness, compassion, and respect. I hope that one day, all military members, veterans, and their families can receive the same support.

Dr. Cheryl Martin—a true frentor, "mentor + friend," who has been a guiding force in reimagining and redesigning healthcare to be a safe and fulfilling place for our healthcare workers.

Dr. Resa E. Lewiss is a frentor in writing, podcasting, and being a changemaker in medicine. Her generosity in sharing advice, making introductions, and listening intently has greatly impacted my development.

Dr. Dan Dworkis is a dear friend and collaborator. He granted my request to be a guest podcast host on his podcast, which gave me the confidence to start my podcast. Podcasting helped me develop the ideas in this book.

Amanda Hill, JD for her suggested edits to this book and all-around support of me personally and professionally.

Seth W. Wiener, Esq. for legal counsel and proofing assistance related to this book.

Erica Bristol, Esq. at Full Circle Business Law, PC for legal services related to publishing this book.

Dr. Michelle Sergel- inspired me to become a simulation educator. Dr. Carmen Spalding, Dr. Joseph Lopreiato and Dr. Alexis Batista for ongoing mentorship and sponsorship in simulation and medical education.

Dr. Dara Kass for her advocacy work that inspires me, and for being a wonderful accomplice.

Dr. Gillian Schmitz for encouraging me to get involved in GSACEP and ACEP and teaching me the power of collective agency.

Dr. Mizuho Morrison—sent me my first podcast microphone and taught me how to podcast.

Dr. Christina Shenvi, The Whole Physicians (Dr. Laura Cazier, Dr. Amanda Dinsmore, Dr. Kendra Morrison), and Dr. Tracy Sanson for their involvement in Revitalize Women Physician Circle and your frentorship. All of you embody what it means to revitalize.

Thank you, Dr. Linda Lawrence, for your mentorship, coaching, and collaboration. I've learned so much from you. Thank you for supporting me in following my heartline.

I want to thank every guest on my podcast. You've expanded my mind and, most importantly, my heart on what is possible in healthcare.

SUGGESTED BOOK CLUB OR GROUP DISCUSSION QUESTIONS

1. What attracted you to your field? Are there new factors that increase your passion and joy in work now?

2. What strategies do you utilize to go from being a (insert profession, e.g., doctor, nurse) to practicing that profession?

3. How do you know if you need to take a break or need support? What signs do you see in others that may suggest they need a break or support?

4. What systems of support are available in your workplace? Are there any gaps you want to address that may enhance mentorship, coaching, peer support, debriefs, etc.? What is an action step towards making that change?

5. The concept of "Just Like Me" networks was discussed. What are some ways that you can increase the diversity of your networks and promote more inclusive workplaces?

6. How does your workplace support women and people from historically underrepresented groups in healthcare? What are some areas for improvement in recruiting, retaining, and promoting women and persons from underrepresented groups?

7. The term resilience has been overused and sometimes used against healthcare workers. What does resilience mean to you? How does an individual think about their resilience in relation to

some of the healthcare system's challenges? For instance, when should someone consider leaving a toxic workplace versus optimizing their resiliency or adaptability to a workplace?

8. Vulnerability is a pathway to connection. How have you authentically shown vulnerability to enhance connection with patients and colleagues?

9. Do you currently experience moral injury? If so, is there a situation you'd like to share with the group? Brainstorm some solutions on how to respond to this situation to advocate for patients and healthcare workers affected by the dynamics contributing to moral injury.

10. Trauma is inherent to working in healthcare. What strategies do you use to process trauma? How do you support others around you to process trauma?

11. The book introduces individual and collective agency. How are you connecting with others at your workplace, professional organizations, and other larger groups to address the challenges that require group effort?

12. What trip did you feel was therapeutic? If you haven't experienced therapeutic travel yet, what place would you like to visit to grow, heal, or learn?

ABOUT THE AUTHOR

Dr. Andrea Austin is a leading emergency physician, simulation educator, and advocate for physician well-being. Firmly believing in the power of a well-being-oriented workforce to deliver superior care, Dr. Austin's work focuses on autonomy, belonging, and competency for healthcare providers. Her pioneering efforts advocate for simulation as a pivotal tool in healthcare education.

As a prior Lieutenant Commander in the United States Navy, her active-duty Navy career included a deployment to Iraq in 2016. She later became the first woman emergency medicine physician stationed at the Navy Trauma Training Center (NTTC) at LA County + USC, one of the busiest trauma centers in the United States. Serving at the forefront of emergency medicine at the NTTC, she trained hundreds of military personnel. As the Director of the Naval Postgraduate's Simulation in Healthcare program, she continues to positively impact the development of educational innovations through the military and VA systems.

Dr. Austin advocates for a supportive healthcare culture. She is committed to improving the culture of healthcare through an emphasis on the well-being of workers, patient safety, and a culture of innovation. She is the host of the *Heartline: Changemaking in Healthcare* podcast.

RESOURCES

[1] Source: https://www.pbs.org/wgbh/nova/doctors/oath_modern.html

[2] Term first coined by Barbara Ehrenreich and John Ehrenreich in 1970, and introduced to me by Dr. Anna Barrett on *Heartline* podcast, episode 25.

[3] The Midlife Unraveling: term coined by Dr. Brené Brown

[4] For a deep dive into moral injury in the medical system, I recommend Dr. Wendy Dean's book, If I Betray these Words.

[5] Porter J, Boyd C, Skandari MR, Laiteerapong N. Revisiting the Time Needed to Provide Adult Primary Care. J Gen Intern Med. 2023;38(1):147-155. doi:10.1007/s11606-022-07707-x

[6] For a deep dive for how AI is and will transform medicine, I recommend: Deep Medicine: How Artificial Intelligence Can Make Healthcare Human Again by Eric Topol

[7] During my midlife unraveling that spurred this book, I relied heavily on Emotional Agility: Get Unstuck, Embrace Change, and Thrive in Work and Life by Susan David to increase my emotional intelligence and embrace emotions as data, not directives.

[8] https://www.mhanational.org/co-dependency

[9] Gartrell NK, Milliken N, Goodson WH 3rd, Thiemann S, Lo B. Physician-patient sexual contact. Prevalence and problems. West J Med. 1992;157(2):139-143.

[10] George Tyndall, U.S.C. Gynecologist Accused of Sex Abuse. Jesus Jiménez. Oct. 5, 2023. The New York Times.

[11] Harbor-UCLA Medical Center director resigns amid doctor's

misconduct litigation by By Anna Dai-Liul. Dec. 16, 2023. https://dailybruin.com/2023/12/16/harbor-ucla-medical-center-director-resigns-amid-doctors-misconduct-litigation. The Daily Bruin

12 The Larry Nassar Case: What Happened and How the Fallout Is Spreading. Christine Hauser and Maggie Astor. Jan. 25, 2018

13 McClain T, Kammer-Kerwick M, Wood L, Temple JR, Busch-Armendariz N. Sexual Harassment Among Medical Students: Prevalence, Prediction, and Correlated Outcomes. Workplace Health & Safety. 2021;69(6):257-267. doi:10.1177/2165079920969402

14 Menon A. Sexism and Sexual Harassment in Medicine: Unraveling the Web. J Gen Intern Med. 2020;35(4):1302-1303. doi:10.1007/s11606-019-05589-0

15 Newman C, Templeton K, Chin EL. Inequity and Women Physicians: Time to Change Millennia of Societal Beliefs. Perm J. 2020;24:1-6. doi:10.7812/TPP/20.024

16 Gettel CJ, Courtney DM, Agrawal P, Madsen TE, Rothenberg C, Mills AM, Lall MD, Keim SM, Kraus CK, Ranney ML, Venkatesh AK. Emergency medicine physician workforce attrition differences by age and gender. Acad Emerg Med. 2023 Nov;30(11):1092-1100. doi: 10.1111/acem.14764. Epub 2023 Jun 23. PMID: 37313983.

17 https://medicineiowa.org/spring-2022/andrea-austin-military-physician-simulation-educator

18 Kalmoe MC, Chapman MB, Gold JA, Giedinghagen AM. Physician Suicide: A Call to Action. Mo Med. 2019;116(3):211-216.

19 The rise of long-distance marriage. The Economist. Dec. 19, 2017. https://www.economist.com/united-states/2017/12/19/the-rise-of-long-distance-marriage

20 Bayazit H, Ozel M, Arac S, Dulgeroglu-Bayazit D, Joshi A.

Posttraumatic Stress Disorder Among Health Care Workers During the COVID-19 Pandemic. J Psychiatr Pract. 2022;28(5):354-361. Published 2022 Sep 1. doi:10.1097/PRA.0000000000000661

[21] Fond G, Fernandes S, Lucas G, Greenberg N, Boyer L. Depression in healthcare workers: Results from the nationwide AMADEUS survey. *Int J Nurs Stud.* 2022;135:104328. doi:10.1016/j.ijnurstu.2022.104328

https://www.ncbi.nlm.nih.gov/pmc/articles/PMC9359895/

[22] They Spent Their Life Savings on Life Coaching by Katie Bishop, Published June 2, 2024, Updated June 7, 2024. https://www.nytimes.com/2024/06/02/business/life-coach-debt-savings.html

[23] Alok Patel and Stephanie Plowman. The Increasing Importance of a Best Friend at Work. August 17, 2022. https://www.gallup.com/workplace/397058/increasing-importance-best-friend-work.aspx

[24] Linzer M, Visser MRM, Oort FJ, Smets EMA, McMurray JE, de Haes HCJM. Predicting and preventing physician burnout: results from the United States and the Netherlands. The American journal of medicine. 2001;111(2):170-175. doi:10.1016/S0002-9343(01)00814-2

[25] Abramson LY, Seligman ME, Teasdale JD. Learned helplessness in humans: Critique and reformulation. Journal of abnormal psychology (1965). 1978;87(1):49-74. doi:10.1037/0021-843X.87.1.4

[26] George AE, Frush K, Michener JL. Developing physicians as catalysts for change. Acad Med. 2013 Nov;88(11):1603-5. doi: 10.1097/ACM.0b013e3182a7f785. PMID: 24072124

[27] Bandura A. Social cognitive theory: An agentic perspective. Annual review of psychology. 2001;52(1):1-26.

doi:10.1146/annurev.psych.52.1.1

[28] https://www.bbc.com/news/world-africa-68769839

https://www.bbc.com/news/world-africa-39271850

[29] More than Simply "Doing Good": A Definition of Changemaker. February,2016.
https://www.evansville.edu/changemaker/downloads/more-than-simply-doing-good-defining-changemaker1.pdf

[30] More than Simply "Doing Good": A Definition of Changemaker. February,2016.
https://www.evansville.edu/changemaker/downloads/more-than-simply-doing-good-defining-changemaker1.pdf

[31] https://www.acep.org/edap

[32] Schäfer, Gráinnea,b; Prkachin, Kenneth M.c; Kaseweter, Kimberley A.c,d; Williams, Amanda C. de Ca,*. Health care providers' judgments in chronic pain: the influence of gender and trustworthiness. PAIN 157(8):p 1618-1625, August 2016. | DOI: 10.1097/j.pain.0000000000000536

[33] Tasca C, Rapetti M, Carta MG, Fadda B. Women and hysteria in the history of mental health. Clin Pract Epidemiol Ment Health. 2012;8:110-119. doi:10.2174/1745017901208010110

[34] Gemzell-Danielsson K, Jensen JT, Monteiro I, et al. Interventions for the prevention of pain associated with the placement of intrauterine contraceptives: An updated review. Acta Obstet Gynecol Scand. 2019; 98: 1500-1513. https://doi.org/10.1111/aogs.13662

[35] https://www.medscape.com/viewarticle/989043

[36] May, C. J., Ostafin, B. D., & Snippe, E. (2020). The relative impact of 15-minutes of meditation compared to a day of vacation in daily life: An exploratory analysis. The Journal of Positive Psychology, 15(2), 278–284. https://doi.org/10.1080/17439760.2019.1610480

[37] Basso JC, McHale A, Ende V, Oberlin DJ, Suzuki WA. Brief, daily meditation enhances attention, memory, mood, and emotional regulation in non-experienced meditators. Behav Brain Res. 2019 Jan 1;356:208-220. doi: 10.1016/j.bbr.2018.08.023. Epub 2018 Aug 25. PMID: 30153464.

[38] https://momastery.com/blog/we-can-do-hard-things-ep-264/

[39] https://momastery.com/blog/we-can-do-hard-things-ep-319/

[40] https://www.gottman.com/blog/the-four-horsemen-the-antidotes/

[41] Iavor Bojinov, Karthik Rajkumar, Guillaume Saint-Jacques, Erik Brynjolfsson, and Sinan Aral. Which Connections Really Help You Find a Job? Harvard Business Review, December 1, 2022. https://hbr.org/2022/12/which-connections-really-help-you-find-a-job

[42] https://hbr.org/2019/08/a-lack-of-sponsorship-is-keeping-women-from-advancing-into-leadership

[43] https://www.andreaaustinmd.com/blog/top-revitalizations-of-2023

[44] Stewart J, Garrido S, Hense C, McFerran K. Music Use for Mood Regulation: Self-Awareness and Conscious Listening Choices in Young People With Tendencies to Depression. Front Psychol. 2019;10:1199. Published 2019 May 24. doi:10.3389/fpsyg.2019.01199

[45] Kramer CK, Leitao CB. Laughter as medicine: A systematic review and meta-analysis of interventional studies evaluating the impact of spontaneous laughter on cortisol levels. PLoS One. 2023;18(5):e0286260. Published 2023 May 23. doi:10.1371/journal.pone.0286260

[46] Xiong RC, Fu X, Wu LZ, et al. Brain pathways of pain empathy activated by pained facial expressions: a meta-analysis of fMRI using the activation likelihood estimation method. Neural Regen Res. 2019;14(1):172-178. doi:10.4103/1673-5374.243722

---

[47] Recalibrate©: Doctor Care an Immersive Development Program for Doctors by Sharee Johnson at Coaching for Doctors.

https://www.coachingfordoctors.net.au/programs/recalibrate-doctor-care/

[48] https://brenebrown.com/podcast/living-big-part-1-of-2/ & https://brenebrown.com/podcast/living-big-part-2-of-2/

[49] https://www.thepsychologylab.com/what-is-polyvagal-therapy & https://www.thepsychologylab.com/what-is-polyvagal-therapy

www.ingramcontent.com/pod-product-compliance
Lightning Source LLC
Chambersburg PA
CBHW061132120626
46546CB00005B/1755